SEX: WOMAN FIRST

How to teach him You come first

A Hollywood Tantra Masseur

Guide to Female Orgasm

The Guide of the Woman Ultimate Pleasure Volume 2

Jean-Claude Carvill

Visit website jeanclaudecarvillbooks.com

Jean-Claude Carvill

Copyright @2012 Jean-Claude Carvill

The material of this book is for entertainment purpose only. The use of this material is not intended as a medical or other health professional service to address your specific personal needs. Readers are encouraged to consult with qualified health care practitioners for diagnosis and treatments. The author does not assume any legal responsibility for the use or misuse of any information contained within. Always consult a competent professional for answers to your specific questions.

All rights reserved. No part of this book may be used or reproduced in any manner whatsoever without written permission except in the case of brief quotations embodied in critical articles and reviews.

To A. for her implicit trust to let love and passion

bringing sparkles to her eyes.

Contents

Introduction 5
Chapter 1   Chakras and Sexual Awakening 16
Chapter 2   The Tantric Breath of Love 32
Chapter 3   Tantric Massage 50
Chapter 4   Anatomy of the Yoni 90
Chapter 5   Romancing the Yoni 108
Chapter 6   Self-Pleasure or Masturbation 137
Chapter 7   Exploring the A-spot and the G-spot 153
Chapter 8   The Fountain of Love: Female Ejaculation 176
Chapter 9   How Women Can Become Multiple Orgasmic 193
Chapter 10   I Lost My Sexuality! How Do I Regain It? 208
Chapter 11   The Tantric Lingam: Anatomy and Pleasuring of the Penis and Male G-spot 223
Chapter 12   The Best Six Sex Positions for a Woman to Achieve Orgasm 246
Chapter 13   Date with Your Lover 254
Chapter 14   Tantra Quickies 264
Chapter 15   Fetishism, Fantasies and Role Playing in the Tantric World 269
Chapter 16   Goodbye and Good Morning 279
Conclusion 289
Glossary 292
Questionnaire 297
About the Author 298

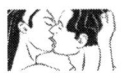

INTRODUCTION

When I gave my very first Tantra massage in 1980, the instructor admonished us sternly, "Remember, you are not allowed to touch any private parts of the person you are massaging. This is a Tantra class, not the privacy of your bedroom." Tantra at the time was only just being introduced in the Western world. The discipline originated in India, as a fundamental part of the mysterious philosophy of Hinduism. We actually knew very little about the sexuality associated with Tantra. At the time it was still pretty taboo!

One day while I was massaging my partner with Tantric devotion, completely dedicated to the appreciation of her wonderful, sensual body, something rather strange happened. I felt her body quivering and shuddering under my hands. I felt her breathing accelerate and I noticed that the lobes of her ears had become reddish. Then her body became utterly tense—but soon relaxed again. No one else could possibly have noticed this happening, as it was barely perceptible. But I knew she had had an orgasm, and I was truly amazed. It had happened so easily! I thought I must have touched an erogenous zone without being aware of it. Once I was finished massaging her, a very stylish English woman, she walked away with a huge smile and told me, "You are very good! Great hands, I needed it badly."

During my next seminar, I had the opportunity to talk to a very beautiful, elegant lady named Narayani, who was taking the course with me. She seemed very confident in her sexuality. Intrigued, I asked her why she had taken this class.

She confessed that she was in a very boring relationship. She loved the man and would never consider leaving him, but she wanted to find out about Tantra. *"My husband is selfish and it often times leads me to feel undesirable. I think the standard situation is that he doesn't know how to complete my pleasure. Most men don't know what they are doing. I also get caught up fulfilling my obligations as a mother that I forget about myself. I want to experience a different and higher level of sexuality and my body shakes a lot and I think I'm at some sexual age peak. I just want to do whatever it is my body is wanting. I have never had man even regular massage me but I don't feel there is anything wrong with this. It's making me kind of resent my husband and I don't want that. It took me until last year to orgasm with my clit and I want to know all about the G-spot. I never knew it existed. I am a little difficult in the orgasm department but I can do it to myself in about 4-5 min on my clit. I really don't know what I want. But my body is screaming at me."* She felt that there was so much more within herself she had not yet discovered; she felt as if she might explode. She went on to say that her husband was too shy, introvert and fragile to come to the class, but that she would go back and share her newfound knowledge with him. She hoped it would bring some excitement back to their bedroom.

As I traveled from Sydney to Hollywood via Pune and Paris, I heard the same complaint over and over again. I settled down in Beverly Hills and became a Hollywood Tantra masseur. Women from all walks of life contacted me, from the White House office to the big screen; I became the darling of the show biz world.

Just yesterday I received an email stating, *"My husband and I have been together for 16 years. We have a wonderful marriage filled with joy from our children. Unfortunately, for reasons I don't completely understand, my husband has no sex drive. The issue began years ago and has progressed to the point where we have no intimate relations at all. Your help would be greatly appreciated."*

Other women have contacted me because they have problems achieving orgasm with their partner. One wrote, "*I've been through several traumas, from rape to abuse. I find that I'm aroused quite a lot but have trouble climaxing with others. I can bring myself to orgasm without a problem, but when someone else is involved, it's not so easy. I'm not really sure what else to say, but if you think you could help, let me know.*" Also, I frequently receive messages of this sort: "*I have orgasm only by clitoral stimulation through masturbation, but I never had an orgasm with my husband.*" I usually reply: "*As long you can achieve orgasm through self-pleasure, there is no reason you cannot do the same with your partner. Relax, breathe, and teach him how to love your body.*" Often, I get this type of emails "*Dear Jean-Claude I think we are missing passion, spontaneity and initiative from my husband because most of the times that we have sex it's been initiated by me. Our sex has become boring and always takes place in our bedroom and always ends up in the same missionary position because it's the only way - that I know of for myself. Our love making just isn't exciting or long-lasting anymore.*" Deborah O.

Everywhere I turn, women are losing the precious connection they have with their partner because he does not understand what the female body craves. Therefore the couple become bored with each other and loses the excitement they shared in the beginning of their relationship. If our relationships between man and woman stay as exciting as the first days , couples would stay together forever. Yet that spark at the beginning can be deepened into a steady flame if a couple gains more knowledge of how their bodies and minds can be intertwined.

The famous erotic Kama Sutra sculptures of the Khajuraho temples in India, built between 950 and 1150 C.E., were the first sex guides ever created. Spiritually, those who practice Tantra seek to contact the divine energy of the universe and channel it within the human body by means of ritual in order to achieve creativity and freedom.

Tantra is the connection of all consciousness, and consciousness is in everything—but especially in sex.

Ever since that first Tantra massage seminar, I have not stopped exploring women's bodies. I have discovered their ultimate and most hidden secrets and the truly magical results of certain special soft caresses. I have learned what happens when these magic and sometime taboo spots become aroused. Once she herself discovers that spot via such innocent touches as having her feet caressed, her lips softly touched, her inner legs kissed softly or her most hidden erogenous zones—like her A-spot—gently stimulated, she blossoms with joy. She feels much lighter and happier. She becomes terribly excited that her body can now give her endless ecstatic pleasures that she has never felt before. Often these women tell me that they feel as if they have come "home" at last. A real, lasting bond is built with their partner.

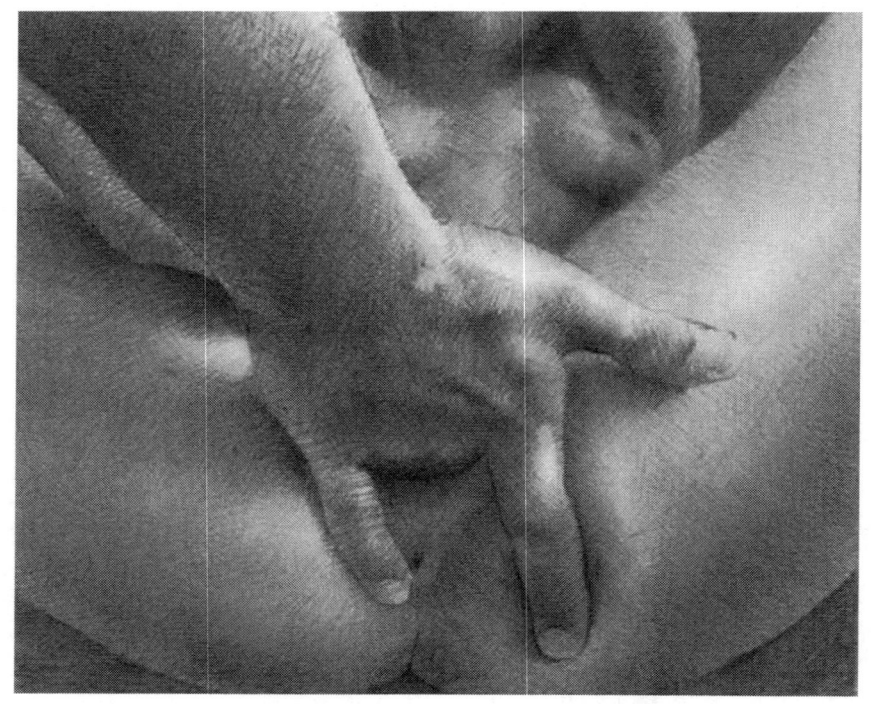

I feel how much sex a woman had and how long it will take for her to squirt

My story and experience is different than others who wrote about the same subject in that I am not a doctor, neither a woman lesbian, a young sexy man, a gigolo, a porn actor, a movie producer, or a famous writer. I worked hard to acquire my knowledge. I am one of the rare or only ones who personally massaged and made ejaculated several hundred women. My experience does not come from books, videos or a few women I met in a bar on Saturday night. You may recall my unusual life story in my last book *The Confession of a Hollywood Tantra Masseur*. Thanks to the feedback on my website left by the women I pleasured, I met women daily, years after years. I finally developed such sensitive fingers that when I do a G-spot massage I feel how much sex a woman have had and how long it will take for her to squirt. (*see drawing: I feel how much sex a woman had and how long it will take for her to squirt*) I wrote that book for you to inherit of my experience and to save time and frustration. This book provides a coaching-based relationship to your sexuality. It helps you explore ways you can teach yourself to have a more joyous, expressive, and confident life of intimacy. Explore this book not from the perspective that you have a problem and need to fix it. Instead, read these pages and wonder what it would mean if you fully experienced and enjoyed your sexuality. Like Jane, who feel so fortunate *"My partners have all made sure I finished first, and when I know I'm not going to I verbalize it and ask them to finish. I've never had a man turn that down. It would show more concern for me and my needs if he stopped and laid with me feeling if I couldn't climax he wouldn't either, but that's more of a romantic idea than anything I'd ever expect."*

I should caution that I am not a doctor. Some sexual concerns have a foundation in physical health, and these are better addressed by a physician. Yet I gave my first Tantric massage 35 years ago, and I have helped so many to strengthen their mind-body relationship. Most likely this book could save your sexual life, marriage or long term relationship.

What does it mean to have a fully alive emotional relationship with your sexual energy? Modern Tantra describes the connections between the pelvis and the heart and other upper chakras. Chakras are the force centers in your body, which receive and transmit energy. While many people don't sense the actual energy flow, they do experience the capacity to connect emotionally and spiritually with one's partner. Many people experience it as the ability to lose control over their minds and bodies in moments of pure surrender while also being fully present with their partner. In this state, a person is able to be fully alive in the act of lovemaking, connected to one's partner emotionally and sensually, while also being fully aware of the experience of pleasure and physical joy in one's own body.

When you read the above description, it sounds wonderful. Why aren't people in this state all the time? Part of the reason is because intimacy is a double-edged sword. To be fully alive during the highs, such as a mind-blowing orgasm, you also have to be willing to participate during the lows. Intimacy is the ability to completely share one's self with one's partner. You cannot hold back the truth of your experiences, both the joyous and the challenging.

Emotional intimacy starts with the mind. You have to be willing to share, with your partner, even to be vulnerable. The power of being naked extends beyond the physical—it equally applies to being exposed emotionally. In the same way you want to touch your partner with your hands, your desire for emotional intimacy can be expressed by sensations of joy, laughter, and even sorrow at certain times. This reaching out to your partner extends in many ways, and if you remain open, the heart/pelvic combination is an extremely powerful one.

When emotional patterns are interfering with sexual expression, you can experience a variety of distressing symptoms. You can feel a loss of desire for your own partner. You may experience a desire for a different partner. You may find you have an inability to achieve an orgasm, erection or to maintain one, or suffer from premature ejaculation. Sex can feel more like a duty, more stressful than fun. A man can become preoccupied with his ability to please his partner, wondering whether he is doing "enough," and then find himself limp. Or he can feel so pressured that he tunes out completely. You would be surprised how often one partner is not fully present during the act of lovemaking.

If you sense these issues are holding you back, here are some questions you can explore to help you start understanding how to overcome them. Remember: Many men forget that taking the risk to be vulnerable actually shows their strength. It takes a lot of courage to acknowledge your anxieties and to be willing to share them with your partner. This can be the first step in moving beyond them.

Think about each of these questions before writing down an answer to them:

1. What happens when you don't feel completely safe being truly intimate with your partner?
2. Where do your thoughts and attention go while having sex?
3. Do you sense that your discomfort arises from this particular relationship or from some unresolved issue in your past?
4. What are your physical responses to anxiety?
5. Do you notice tension anywhere in your body?
6. What feelings emerge when you make eye contact with your partner during sex?

By answering these questions, you begin gathering information about yourself—and what makes you hold back. Once you answer them honestly, you can get at the root of the problems. Ask yourself these questions, and again, really think about them:

1. What allows you to feel safe with another person?
2. What does a strong connection to another person feel like for you?
3. Where is your awareness when you're experiencing truly spectacular sex?
4. What were the three best intimate (sexual or otherwise) experiences of your life, and what specifically made them so wonderful?
5. What about intimacy is important for you?
6. What do you need to ask of your partner?
7. What does it feel like to be aware of your partner's reactions while being fully aware of your own body at the same time?

Here's an exercise you can do to discover your sexual values. Imagine your absolute ideal sexual encounter. Describe everything about it: the place you're in, the time of day, what you and your partners are (or are not) wearing, how you are touching each other, and also the energy that is present between you. Go into as much imaginative detail as possible, and remember that this is your absolute ideal. When you are finished imagining this encounter, write down everything. Then make a list of all of your descriptions. Which 10 are the most important to you? What will you commit to doing that will bring all 10 of these elements to the act next time you make love with your partner?

Ultimately, this area of exploration can lead you into a deeper intimate relationship with your partner. At the same time it will increase your capacity to enjoy your own body. Once you acknowledge your potential anxieties, you can manage them. You can unlock of the barriers to trust and expressing your emotions.

The guide you are about to read focuses your mind on your body's actions. There are no goals in Tantra, because what you do is your goal. You need to be living fully in the present, and the precious union with your partner is all that matters. You do not have to please. Simply follow your instincts, and you will find you are dancing with your sensuality.

This book will teach you how a woman can access her magical spots so that they bring her the ultimate sexual pleasure in a spiritual and harmonious manner. You may discover that sucking your toes or being licked under your feet brings tremendous pleasure. (*see drawing: Sucking your toes or being licked under your feet brings tremendous pleasure*) Maybe the back of your knees is the source of your greatest pleasure. You may discover that having your nipples licked the right way at the right time is the source of your first multiple orgasm. This guide also shows how a man can become a master in the art of making love. In the end, you can bring back the love and joy that should be present in the bedroom. Any one of the chapters in *Sex-Woman First* may open the door to the orgasm you have been waiting for all your life. Or, you may find you can improve the orgasms you already have, making them more explosive. Ultimately, you will have multiple orgasms.

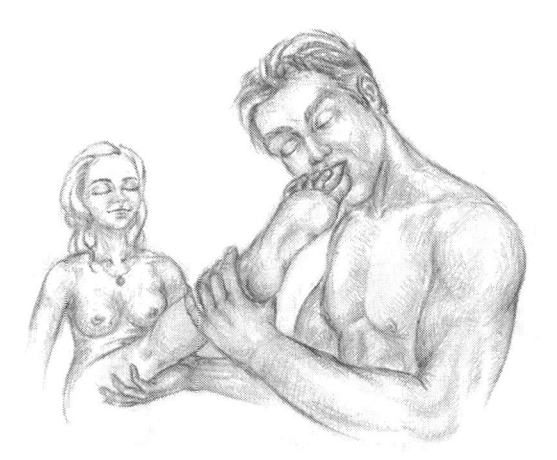

Sucking your toes or being licked under your feet brings tremendous pleasure

14 Sex: Woman First

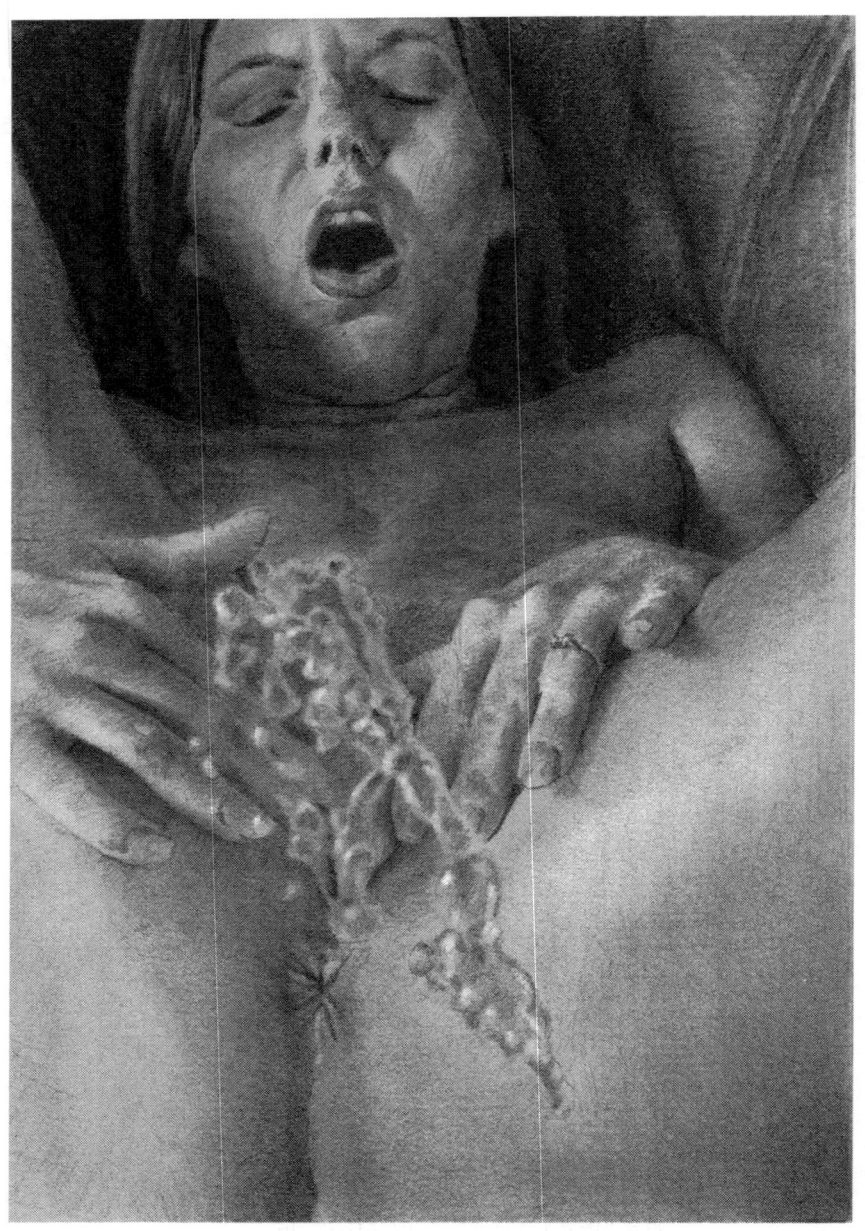

You may even have a female ejaculation

You may even have a female ejaculation, squirting, ending one of these passionate nights soaking the bed of your *Amrita*. (*see drawing: You may even have a female ejaculation*). Finally, each chapter features a clear outline of its contents and benefits. There are also suggested exercises to help you regain trust in yourself and to bring that smile back to your face.

For a couple, Tantra explores the union and communication with your partner. Solo, Tantra shows the way to freedom from suppression, becoming who you really are sexually. When you become sexually conscious, you can achieve your ultimate pleasure.

I am inviting you to share my journey, to realize that foreplay is as important and even more than penetration. From today you can break out of your state of routine, and approach sex as an art, you can pleasure your Goddess with the same passion as an artist who paints a great canvas. Sex is an art and you are the artist who give pleasure to your partner. Because you are going to become a great lover, and nothing in the world can create more pleasure than an orgasm and you are going to be the one who is going to give that greatest pleasure to your Goddess or your God. Finally, you too can be the lover of your dreams.

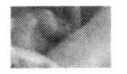

CHAPTER 1

Chakras and Sexual Awakening

It was sometime in January, a new year had just begun, and I often found myself, like many others, contemplating my life and past achievements and wondering what the future would bring. Although sometimes life seems to have its own pace, heedless of where I wanted to go or how fast I wanted to get there, somehow, when I look back, it all makes sense. Looking back at the path life had set me on, and seeing the main knots where all things came together, it seems that I was destined for Tantric massage.

One of those crucial turning points came when I was in India, sitting on a bench near the Ganges River. It was there that I met a very special person, Dr. Gandharva Mavulykvyas, who later became a dear friend of mine. It was him who taught me about Indian perceptions of body and soul, about the way energy flows through our bodies, and how this energy can be transformed and passed from one person to another. Dr. G. Mavulykvyas also told me about chakras and how they can be opened through Tantra.

This is how Dr. G. Mavulykvyas explained Tantra to me: "*In the Hindu and Buddhist cultures, Tantra has been used for ages. Tantra is not about sex; it is a way to soothe your inner self by focusing energy on certain parts of your body. Our body has different chakras (see drawings: "Men Chakra" and "Woman Chakra") In Sanskrit, the word chakra means "a moving wheel." The body is said to have seven main chakra levels located near the spine. These chakras are the channels of universal life, which motivate and energize us to live healthy lives. When a person experiences pain at a personal or emotional level, Tantra can help. It can unblock the energies trapped inside the body at the closest chakra. A Tantric massage specialist will help you understand the complications in your chakras and help you overcome and get rid of these problems for life."*

This information helped me a lot, years later, with one of my clients, Giselle, who had an unusual story:

Giselle had been molested at a young age and was unable to work past her sexual issues, which were a direct result of that incident. She needed her chakras opened more than anything. My intention, when she requested Tantric massage, was to open Giselle's chakras and heal the blockage within her soul by whatever means it took.

I gave Giselle a task to watch videos about Tantric massage on YouTube and let me know if she thought Tantric massage might help her. When she called me back, all she said was, "Interesting. I watched the chakras massage on YouTube. It looks sensual and relaxing, and also sexually stimulating. I definitely have some blockages in life. Most are not sexual but spiritual in nature. I would like to connect my spiritual side with my sensual side, to feel trust and love, if it's possible."

"Even though the problems may not be sexual in nature," I told Giselle, "Tantric massage can relieve all kinds of emotional and spiritual blockages. Massage that balances the chakras will open a great source of sexual energy."

Giselle's home was immaculate, and she was ready, greeting me at the door with only a muumuu on her ample body. "I hope you don't mind my greeting you practically naked," she said.

She willingly undressed without being asked and placed herself on her back on the bed as I removed various oils and other soothing liquids from my small case.

I used a very sensual and soft Tantric massage in order to help Giselle to get in touch with her body and raise her inner Goddess. Her desire to explore and heal was inspiring—and so she did, without prejudice or fear.

The Chakras

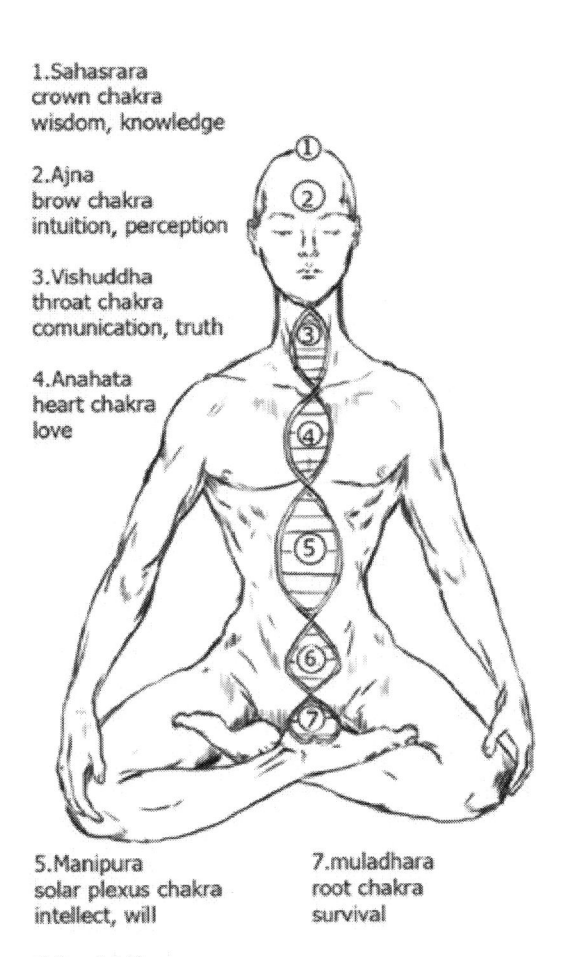

1. Sahasrara
crown chakra
wisdom, knowledge

2. Ajna
brow chakra
intuition, perception

3. Vishuddha
throat chakra
comunication, truth

4. Anahata
heart chakra
love

5. Manipura
solar plexus chakra
intellect, will

6. Svadhisthana
sacral chakra
joy, sexuality

7. muladhara
root chakra
survival

Men Chakra

The Chakras

1. Sahasrara(violet)
crown chakra
wisdom, knowledge

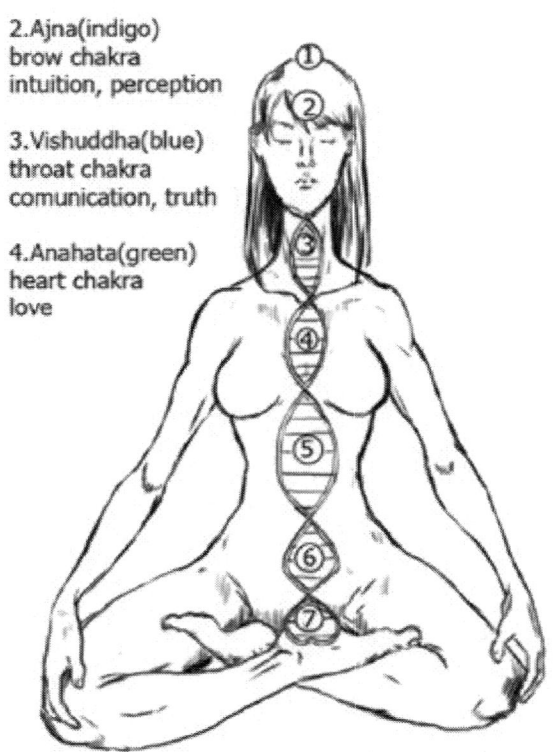

2. Ajna(indigo)
brow chakra
intuition, perception

3. Vishuddha(blue)
throat chakra
comunication, truth

4. Anahata(green)
heart chakra
love

5. Manipura(yellow)
solar plexus chakra
intellect, will

6. Svadhisthana(orange)
sacral chakra
joy, sexuality

7. muladhara
root chakra
survival

Women Chakra

In addition to balancing the energy flow between mind, body, emotions, and spirit, the chakras also illustrate some of the differences between male and female sexual energy in a way that is useful and practical. (*see drawings: Men Chakra and Woman Chakra*)

For many women, men appear to have a certain sexual advantage, since their satisfaction is quick, easy, and uncomplicated. Once a woman learns the many different ways she has to enjoy orgasmic sexual pleasure, she no longer considers herself lucky when she gets a single orgasm. Her many sources of sexual pleasure are awakened and she knows how to energize and activate each of them, giving her a wondrous appreciation for her complex and beautiful body.

As a woman, you may come more slowly to sexual excitation and satisfaction than a man; that is true. One reason for this is that you have so many more components of your sexual anatomy that contribute to your pleasure. Some components are responsive naturally with the correct physical stimulation, while others are more responsive when you have an orchestra of sensual instruments playing together.

Tantric sexual pleasure is more accessible when the chakras are unblocked and balanced, particularly the primal chakras. Certain chakra exercises, along with techniques for couples and singles, enable each woman to uncover and empower all of her sensual, emotional, and physical features to achieve complete sexual pleasure and orgasm.

The first and most important lesson is that every woman is different and has unique perceptions and desires. In Tantra, full female sexual potential is achieved through gentle and loving touch based on personal preferences, and then expanding on these when a woman is ready. There is no rush to accomplishment but, rather, a savoring of each step of increased female pleasure along the journey.

Many times both men and women erroneously think that a woman's full pleasure is impossible because some obstacle lies in the way. What they do not know is that a woman's body is designed head to toe for sensual and sexual pleasure. Tantric massage will awaken all of the possibilities, one by one. Take what works for you and use it with love, appreciation, and joy.

Importance of Unblocking and Breathing Exercises

A woman's misconceptions about her bodily functions, especially the sexual organs, and her own mental and emotional reservations often contribute to a combined failure of stimulus and response. She may feel pleasure during foreplay or intercourse, for example, but find that it is insufficient to arouse her to orgasm.

Email received *"Dear Jean-Claude, Lately I feel not satisfied with just one orgasm. I believe that it is because I am blocked in my chakras. The last partner I took to bed did not help me to get aroused enough and then after he came from my oral on him, he left. Men are so selfish" Kimberly G.*

Breathing exercises and chakra meditations are not just vague suggestions for getting in touch with ourselves, but concrete ways for a woman to read her body for pleasurable stimulation and make sure that all the pleasure signals are fully functioning. Although you might go water or snow skiing only at certain times of the year, you can't let your body get out of condition during the off season and then expect things to go well once the weather changes. Likewise, if you invest little in your sexual readiness, you will find that your body fails to respond when you want it to.

For men, things seem to be much simpler, because their bodies are built in a way that allows them to be ready for sex in a very short amount of time from the beginning of the sexual stimulation. Apparently, this happens because, in prehistoric times, men had to be ready to procreate fast and then go hunting, and their easy-to-arouse nature has endured.

For a woman, things are not quite that simple, because a woman may often allow her mind to wander to her family, to her workload, to lists and errands, to relationships with friends, to an upcoming event or past trauma, to her home, to her body flaws, and on and on. These thoughts deprive her of the moment she is experiencing and of her potential for intimacy and ecstasy, so her libido diminishes and her arousal and sensuality also go down, just when she needs them the most.

Examining our chakras is a great way to determine where we are out of balance physically, mentally, emotionally, and spiritually. It is like a checkup for your entire being. You can seek the experience of a Tantric masseur to detect imbalances in the chakras and help with blockages, but this is very much a self-help healing area as well, and I will gladly show you how to do this for yourself.

The important message here is not that every mental or physical problem has a sexual solution but that, regardless of any other troubling physical or mental issues, a woman can find blissful sexual contentment in a variety of ways and that true sexual pleasure itself is very healing.

The meditation at the end of this chapter will help you to transfer the beneficial effects of your awakened chakras into your sexual experience, making it completely unforgettable and whole. It will also help to keep your mind in the present moment and all of your life forces flowing freely through your body during sex. This way your sexuality will expand into your entire being, and it will feel wonderful.

Detecting Blockage and its Causes

Chakra work helps a woman to balance all of her sexual elements holistically. Gradually, she trains each chakra to contribute harmoniously to her energy flow and achieve a wondrous orgasm through her choice of oral, manual, penile, or other stimulation.

Each of your seven chakra energy centers can be underactive, balanced, or overactive. An overactive chakra generally is attempting to compensate for one or more that is underactive, so the simplest way to restore balance is to stimulate the weak chakras. As these begin to function more fully, the over-activity in others will diminish.

The specific chakra details are much less important than your own intuitive sense and perceptions. Therefore I want you to take in the information below while avoiding the urge to "take inventory" or to "diagnose and repair." Energy is intended to flow through the chakras, from one in to the other, from the ground to the sky and back, so don't focus too much on particulars; just try to visualize any hot (active) or cold (sluggish) spots or congestion (may be perceived as one feeling meeting an opposite feeling) while doing the meditation exercise. With practice, you can increase your energy flow when and where it is most needed.

Of the seven main chakras, it is believed that the first three, moving from bottom to top, are related to physical needs, financial comfort, basic relationships, and sexual pleasure, while the next four, continuing upward, are related to spiritual needs such as love, creativity, and so on.

The Three Physical Chakras

Root (Muladhara): This most primal chakra at the base of the spine governs basic instinctual elements of physical safety, security, and survival. Weakness or blockage arising from continued disconnection to earth elements appears as lack of energy, listlessness, withdrawal, or a "cold fish" response to touch. The opposite problem is sexual aggressiveness or manipulative behavior.

Sacral (Swadhisthana): The belly or sacral chakra below the navel is most closely aligned with the physical aspect of sexuality in women, but also extends into emotional issues and is associated with feelings such as guilt, shame, blame, and difficulty with intimacy or giving and receiving physical love.

Solar Plexus (Manipura): Located below the wishbone area of the chest, the solar plexus—sexually speaking—is the region associated with issues of control, struggles of will, self-esteem, and vulnerability to the opinions of others. These feelings can internalize in a variety of organs, resulting in distressing physical manifestations. Unblocking here can help women feel less conflicted about experiencing sexual pleasure.

These physical chakras are gifts from Mother Earth and our connection to it. Strengthen them to become more grounded and confident in the physical nature of your sexuality and more self-assured about every aspect of your being as a vital, sensual creature, relaxed and energized by her erotic nature and its pleasures. Blockage generally hinders appreciation, expression, and sharing of these physical energies.

The Four Spiritual Chakras

Heart (Anahata): This is the transformative chakra; the energy center of unconditional love, both given and received, and the ability to transform negative emotions into positive ones. Blockage manifests as unresolved emotional conflict or pain, lack of compassion for self or others, inability to express nurturing, warmth, and kindness, and may cause others to perceive you as distant, aloof, or cold.

Throat (Vishudha): This is the expression chakra. Located about an inch above the root of your neck, it helps you express your feelings, communicate your desires, and socialize verbally. Blockage manifests physically as a sore throat and emotionally as loneliness, as well as the feeling that you are being misunderstood, and/or lack spontaneity and authenticity in your speech.

Third Eye (Ajna): This is the ESP chakra. It is located in the center of your forehead, about ½-inch above the spot between your eyebrows. This is responsible for intuition, premonition, and a special sensitivity to spiritual events. Blockage manifests through lack of a spiritual side and missed opportunities in your life.

The Crown (Sahasrara): Located in the middle of the top of your head. When open, it facilitates access to a higher understanding of the world and helps you detach yourself from daily problems. Blockage manifests as anxiety, excessive fear of death, and preoccupation with having basic necessities.

It is in the Anahat region that we work to balance physical and spiritual energy, heal heart scars, and exchange loving energy with the universe. Blockage in this region prevents the flow of energy between the physical and spiritual (psychic) chakras, such that deep contentment in sexual relationships and sexual pleasure is hindered.

Because it is believed that, in meditation, energy comes from above and enters the body through the crown chakra, gently flowing onward to the rest of the chakras, until the primal chakras are also unblocked and awakened, that is how the meditation exercise is organized. This will enable full opening of all chakras and restoration of energy flow, thereby letting universal energy pass through completely and producing a state of harmony.

Chakra Opening and Alignment Exercises for Self-Healing

Many of the finest healers are those who use intuitive methods to open and align chakras. Intuition is ideal for purposes of female self-healing as well, since women are naturally intuitive and inclined to be quite aware of their general body functioning.

To begin, we will use a simple but powerful meditation exercise to adjust the chakras, and in the next chapter we will follow this up with breathing exercises to complete the cleansing and restoration of energy flow. It is advantageous to do these outdoors where your feet actually touch the earth, but work with what you have and can do. Loose-fitting comfortable clothes can be helpful, as is a chair, but you may sit, stand, or lie on the floor, ground, or mat, and wear whatever you like.

Until you have some experience meditating, avoid discomfort and distractions if possible, but the real power of meditation arises from your intention, not from your positions or accessories. This means that you can perform all or part of your meditations when and where you choose, even in small blocks of time. You can combine these with a morning walk, watering the garden, or kneading bread. Your intention is everything as the boundless energy of the universe is yours if you choose to share in it. After all, you are the energy, as are we all. Relax and enjoy this meditation exercise:

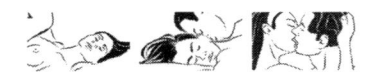

Chakra Exercise

Find a quiet space free of distraction, just for you. The opening of the chakras will help to free you. Take a deep breath and visualize the energy of white light all around you.

- Concentrate on the crown chakra just above your head; visualize a colorful pink flower—a lotus, or a rose—gently moving toward it and opening. Feel purple light going through the center flower, entering into your crown, and moving though your body.

- Visualize the flower floating toward the third-eye chakra. As the flower opens, indigo light showers the center of the flower, flowing into the third eye; opening and clearing blockages. You may feel the energy working its way from the third eye through your body.

- Shift concentration to the throat chakra. Envision the lotus flower opening up and allowing soft blue rays of light to progress into the center of the flower and into the throat chakra. Feel the light flowing through the throat and flowing through you.

- As the focal point becomes the heart chakra, feeling emotional is common. The flower seems to be drawn to the heart chakra. The flower opens, and you experience luminous white and purple lights drawn to the center, entering your heart gently but powerfully.

- Guiding your attention to the solar plexus, envision a warm-colored flower opening as a stream of white light moves toward the center and continues to the entrance of the third chakra, cleansing and empowering all of the organs behind the navel.

- As the attention moves down to the sacral chakra, perceive a warm-colored flower; as the light flows through the chakra, notice sensations from the navel down to the groin.

- As you get closer to the ground, visualize all the light collecting all the blockages, moving down to the base chakra. See the light move down though the base chakra, down the legs, and into the ground.

Motivational Moment

You have taken a new step to understanding how your body uses energy, what the seven chakras are, and how you can open them through meditation.

Most importantly, you have learned a new technique for drawing in and expanding primal sexual energy to use and enhance your energy flow in order to experience orgasm. Also, by opening the sacral chakra, which is the root of sexuality, you can increase your ability to produce multiple orgasms, and experience the wonders of Tantric sex.

Note About Chakras and Sexual Awakening

Chapter One encouraged us to be aware of our seven chakras, especially the primal chakras related to female sexual pleasure, and gave basic instructions for opening, unblocking, and aligning the chakras. Also, a simple but powerful chakra meditation has been provided, to aid with the opening of the chakras and improve orgasmic ability.

Changing our sexual habits has never been easy. Many people find that keeping track of progress helps them to stay motivated and become more open to the experience. I invite you to fill in this log to keep a record of your results.

Some people may do the exercises of each chapter in sequence; others may work on exercises from several chapters simultaneously or at different times. It is recommended that you do all of the exercises (from any chapter) several times a week. Although the log here is for eight weeks only, you will certainly be encouraged by your personal results.

1. Which of these chakras did you open this week: Root, Sacral, Solar Plexus, Heart, Throat, Third Eye, Crown?

2. What change do you want to see in yourself spiritually and sexually: for instance, courage, trust, growth, become a woman, the new me, forgiveness, confidence, letting go of the past, surrender to the present?

3. How do you feel about your own sexuality now that you have done these exercises: for example, beauty, sunshine, regret, assertiveness, enjoyment, pleasure, courage, trust, guilt, benefit?

4. On a scale of 1 to 10, with 10 the maximum, how have these exercises improved the quality of your orgasm(s)?

	1	2	3	4
Week 1				
Week 2				
Week 3				
Week 4				
Week 5				
Week 6				
Week 7				
Week 8				

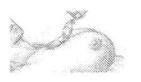

CHAPTER 2

The Tantric Breath of Love

Teagan had been a little vague about the logistics of our meeting. "Wait for me on the corner of Grant and 10th," she said. "Call me when you arrive…the numbers are hard to see from the street." I did as she asked, parking my car and finding a secluded spot to stand, where I could observe the street. Hands dug into my pockets, I waited, trying not to look like I was loitering with intent.

I was starting to think she wouldn't show up when, suddenly, a pair of cool hands came from behind me to cover my eyes. When I tried to turn to see who was there, the hands stayed firm, and their owner swung around with me, staying out of sight.

I laughed, knowing that this must be Teagan. "Are you Jean-Claude?" said a female voice, without even a hint of a smile apparent in its tone.

"Yes, Teagan, I'm Jean-Claude."

"Then follow me."

She was more beautiful than my imaginings. Her sandy hair and even features were quirked by an endearingly childlike gap between her two front teeth and curious green eyes. She smiled at me with an ingenuous openness, and my heart swelled in my chest.

We entered in her small but comfortable apartment, and while I sat on a sofa, she brought me a cup of green tea. She explained why she called me:

"Like many women my age, I have spent many years raising children, working and generally not doing much for myself. But the past couple of years I have awakened to find there is much out there for me to experience and enjoy. I have become much more aware of myself physically and sexually, and would like to continue to expand that knowledge. I have difficulty concentrating on the sensations of my body, because I worry my partner is getting tired or bored because my climax is taking so long. Also, my mind is more engaged in the experience you described on your web site: 'Breathing techniques and awareness of circulating the sexual energy ... to redirect some of the intense arousal energy away from the clitoris and up to the brain and the rest of the body, thus enhancing the capacity for pleasure ... thus stimulation and redirecting the aroused chi (energy) can further enhance the orgasmic experience.'"

"Or, to put it another way, I want to be more focused and not distracted. But I was taught as a child to suppress emotions. I was made to feel that many of my feelings should not be shared. Not necessarily just sexual feelings. But that I shouldn't openly express my deeper feelings."

"In short, I am asking you to come to teach me everything about any breathing techniques that will allow me to have a better orgasm and even multiple orgasms."

Teagan proved to be eager to learn everything. It was like she was trying to fill a void that she has been struggling with for so many years. She was getting in touch with her femininity and her sensuality, and she was becoming increasingly curious. Soon, Teagan learned to relax and increase her pleasure through the use of breathing techniques, and she blossomed beautifully.

In Tantra breathing is to sex as sunshine is to a garden. Breathing is something you do to enhance your own sexual pleasure, and it is a gift to share with your partner. Breathing is an affirmation that you are fully alive and lovingly exchanging energy with the universe around you, inhaling all of its creativity and generosity. Breathing will allow you to respond equally generously with your whole self engaged, your heart filled with joy, and your body surging to release the fluids of love again and again.

When a woman comes to me for Tantric massage, she may be seeking assistance for a variety of sexual difficulties including recovery from previous sexual trauma, physical or mental abuse, rejection or doubts about her ability to achieve an orgasm or to ever fully enjoy it as she yearns to or simply looking for a deeper satisfaction that only purely carnal pleasure. If you as a man can sense that in your partner don't miss it, she will be deeply impress.

Email received "Dear *Jean-Claude, I am searching for something, and I don't know what it is, but I know there is a higher energy or life force from which to live. Tantra, I think, is part of that. I can honestly say I've never had a deeply satisfying sensual exchange with a man. I love sex, but sex is just sex. I'm looking for a deeper experience that will give me more insight into who I am as a woman. I know there is a sexual energy within me that has never been woken up, and I can't seem to do it on my own. I'm a deep, intelligent, passionate woman. I have physical awareness, and I love to be active in/with my body."* Princess Nina

She may have heard that some women are able to enjoy long, satisfying orgasms, multiple orgasms, and even female ejaculation, as well as finding refreshment, energy and peace in their sex lives, but her own sex life seems to be lacking in the aspect she desires most. If she is without a partner, she may not feel confident in her ability to provide her own self pleasure and sexual release.

Tantric sexuality is about finding the techniques and practices that bring each person alive sexually in a manner that nourishes and expands. The breathing exercises presented here will help to establish an automatic connection between mind, body and spirit and dissolve those elements that are blocking your ecstatic orgasmic capacity. You will learn to literally breathe your way into an orgasm (and another and another) and to give and receive sexually with a passionate and open heart.

Breathing defines your life, marking both its beginning and end, and must constantly feed every cell of your body. Breathing is a natural sexual elixir. Learn these simple breathing techniques, and remember to use them, so that you get the full benefit of the Tantric sexuality lessons I will teach. Because breathing is so important, I've given it its own chapter, right here at the beginning of this book. It is that important.

Foreplay and Orgasm

Breathing is vital to stimulating foreplay and achieving orgasm. Maintaining arousal without breathing is like trying to achieve orgasm after a doctor has numbed your pleasure spots with Novocain, yet I encounter this phenomenon over and over again when I work with women through massage.

When nearing orgasm, many women unconsciously begin to hold their breath. Instead of heightening sexual response, stopping the breath effectively deadens it. It is not uncommon for a woman to wonder if she is frigid when she begins to build to a climax and then, suddenly, feels her arousal beginning to fade—yet improper breathing technique may be the sole source of the problem.

Breasts, genitals, skin, and pleasure spots all become more receptive and responsive when fully oxygenated and fed by a lively supply of fresh blood. The breathing exercises shared here will provide this and should also be used to help clear the mind of negative thoughts and distractions.

The time to prepare for utilizing your breathing to either revitalize or relax is long before any sexual moment. You can practice and repeat as often as needed, whether you have five minutes or twenty. With practice, you will be comfortable and prepared and know exactly how to direct your breathing to encourage orgasm and heighten pleasure.

The Nirvana Dance: Breathing and Moving for Better Orgasms

The Nirvana Dance is one of the best exercises for achieving a better orgasm. If you were to read only one paragraph in this whole book, I would want it to be the one that follows, which describes a wonderful exercise that will surely improve your sex life and overall relationship with your partner!

The Nirvana Dance is done lying down on your back on a gym ball. It involves your breathing, your movement, and your voice—one at the time and then all together—while you let go and dream of experiencing the best lovemaking you can imagine. If you don't have a gym ball, you can use a swing seat made with a bed sheet attached from your ceiling or something else. I trust your imagination (*see drawing: The Nirvana Dance is done lying down on your back on a gym ball*)

When you are having sex, your body can easily become strained, and you may lose control of your breath, which becomes short and shallow. What you may not realize is that breathing and the motions your body makes set the frame for an orgasmic sexual experience, so it is very important to know how to move, breathe, and lead your whole body into the experience.

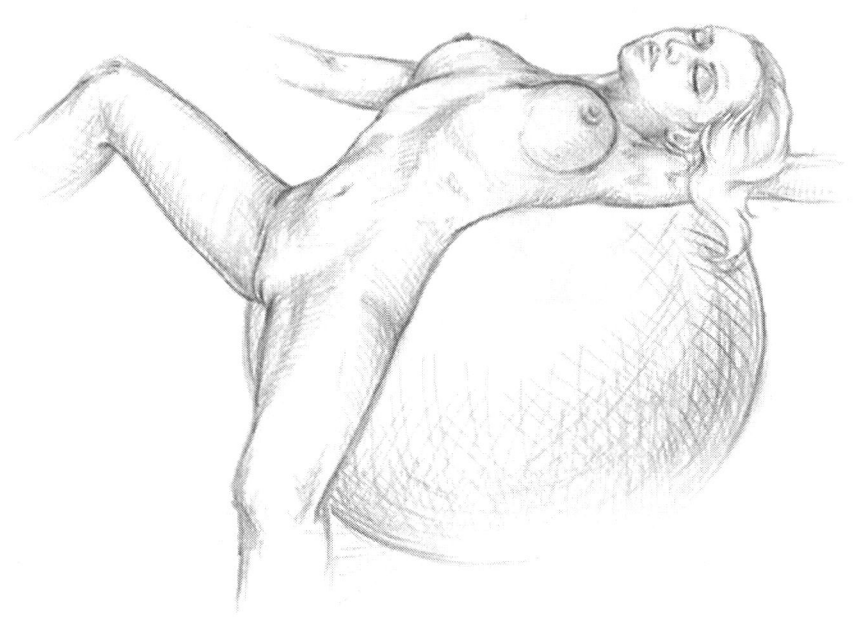

The Nirvana Dance is done lying down on your back on a gym ball

Of course, there are things that sometimes stop us from fully participating in the sexual experience and make us block our reactions. Often, women that I have met during Tantric massage speak about their fear. It might seem illogical to be afraid of a pleasurable experience, but if you have been raised in a strict and conservative environment, you might recognize and understand the mental blockages that can keep a woman from experiencing pleasure, orgasm and multiple orgasms during sex. These same blockages dictate to the body, telling it not to move, to become stiff, and to take short and shallow breaths.

Some of the experiences that could cause a woman to subconsciously block herself from experiencing an orgasm include:

- **Interactions and role-models**: Much of the time, women who struggle to have orgasms speak about having been raised in a very conservative family, with strict rules and no open doors to authentic communication. In some cases, all of their questions about sexuality were treated with silence, or they were sent the message, not necessarily spoken aloud, that sexual pleasure is only for prostitutes. In other families, the prevailing attitude might have been that a sophisticated, well-raised woman only lies still and silent during sex, to fulfill her marital duties. Exposure to these messages over time causes many women to become frigid; in other words, they do not enjoy sex and may see it as a chore they have to do for their husbands.

- **Religion**: If a woman has had a very open and healthy relationship with her family during childhood, but later in life chooses a very restrictive religion, she could inhibit her ability to experience orgasm or feel pleasure during sex—basically by absorbing the same negative attitudes some people experience in childhood.

- **Traumatic Events**: If a woman has been raped or abused, she might come to see intercourse as something painful and disgusting and she will reject her partner, even if she loves him on a conscious level.

- **Self-image:** A woman's inhibitions and negative opinions about her body could stop her from going with the flow and experiencing a whole-body sexual pleasure.

- Alongside psychotherapy to break these types of mental patterns, certain exercises and techniques may be used to help open and relax your body and prepare for a fulfilling sexual experience.

Breathing is one of the two main techniques, along with awakening the blocked chakras, that open the gate to better orgasms. When we are focused on something, we sometimes forget to breathe properly. This usually is a bad thing to do, but during sex it is even worse! Breathing oxygenates the blood; oxygenated blood travelling through the body means more sensitive organs, and thus more intense orgasms.

Still, controlling your breathing probably is the last thing you think of during sex. This is why, through exercise, you teach your body how to breathe and move, so that, during sex, your body will just know what to do, and things will come naturally, while you focus on the pleasure.

Orgasm is an almost reflexive function in which mind and body are equally involved. If you learn how to set the frame for an orgasm, your body will follow and so will orgasm¾without intercourse or any other sexual stimulation, just by breathing and moving your body.

I call it The Nirvana Dance. Different cultures have a similar names, such as the Tahitian dance, belly dancing, and more recently, dirty dancing. You can practice these exercises on your own at first, until you master your breathing techniques. Then you can introduce them to your partner, as a preparation for intercourse, or you could do some on your own and some with your partner. This breathing will increase your level of intimacy, and help you synchronize during sex in order to achieve better orgasms.

Nirvana Dance Part 1: Breathing

- Deep Abdominal Breathing
    1. Use a gym ball to sit up straight and relaxed.
    2. Put one hand on your pelvis and the other on your abdomen, with your fingers spread to your sternum.
    3. Focus on inhaling, and let your chest fill completely with air.

4. Next, focus on exhaling and let all of the air out of your lungs, until you feel your tummy getting closer to your spine.

5. Repeat 15 times.

- Breath Retention

    1. Lie on your back. (You could also use a gym ball under your shoulders and back, and support your weight with your legs).

    2. Put your hands in the same position as before: one on your pelvis, one on your abdomen.

    3. Gently inhale through your nose, retaining the air just as long as it feels comfortable, without feeling the need to gasp for air.

    4. Exhale slowly, focusing your attention on your chest becoming empty and the sound of the air coming out of your mouth.

    5. Repeat 15 times.

Nirvana Dance Part 2: Moving Your Body

- Move Your Pelvis

    1. Lie on your back, and keep your legs on a gym ball, with your knees bent at 90 degrees.

    2. Place your hands on your pelvis and abdomen, just as in the breathing exercises.

    3. Using the breath-retention technique, press your buttocks into the floor while inhaling.

    4. When you exhale, lift your pelvis from the ground.

    5. Repeat these movements, experimenting with the speed of your motion and breathing, until you feel you can perfectly synchronize your breathing with your motion.

- Move Your Chest

    1. Lie on your back with hands alongside your body.

    2. Inhale slowly, and lift your chest.

    3. Then exhale slowly, and push your chest down.

    4. The objective is to synchronize your breathing with the motion of your chest. Once you can do this, you can move on to the next step.

- Combine Pelvis and Chest Movement

    1. After you have mastered the pelvis and chest movement techniques individually, combine them.

    2. When you inhale, lift your chest while pushing down your pelvis.

    3. Retain your breath a little.

    4. When you exhale, lift your pelvis while pushing down your chest.

    5. Repeat, going slowly at first, and then as fast as you would like, until you become more and more aroused. After some practice, you could even have an orgasm just by moving and breathing in this way.

Nirvana Dance Part 3: Exercising Your Voice

I often get e-mails from women who write to me that they want to let go, even wish to learn to speak dirty, to follow their body and lose control. This means that they never lose control while conscious, because of the fear that they will feel vulnerable, get hurt if they open their heart and body, or do something "inappropriate." If you feel the same, these exercises are a great way to practice losing control in a safe environment, especially if you practice them alone. With no one to see or hear you, you are completely safe, so put your whole body into the experience.

Most women use the voice naturally during sex; they scream, they whisper, they share naughty thoughts. Some are completely quiet during intercourse. It is important to use your voice when you do the breathing and motion exercises, at first by whispering and then letting your voice get louder. As you move your body faster, your voice will follow the rhythm. Give voice to everything you are thinking, no matter how silly, dirty, or completely innocent it might seem at first. Whatever works for you is good—just go for it.

Use your imagination. Think of the best orgasm you have ever had, and start to imitate the motions and breathing you used then. Multiply this by 10, and focus on that volume of motion and breathing. When you prepare your body for the best orgasm of your life, both your mind and body will follow and provide a mind-blowing, body shaking climax.

Because you are unique, your motions and rhythm will vary. Do not worry; experiment and find your own pace. Some women also use rotation of the pelvis, keeping their legs on the gym ball for more support. Also, the idea is to pay attention to your body and follow it. If you feel the need to go faster or slower, then do that. If you feel the need to change your position, do that too. You could also try the postures used in hatha yoga. A very helpful one for your breathing and sexual energy is the Cat Asana—the posture of the cat—so named because you imitate the motions of a cat when it is stretching after a rest:

1. Sitting on your knees and hands, use both breathing and motion to increase your sexual energy.

2. When you inhale, keep your butt up and your spine arched to the inside.

3. When you exhale, arch your spine to the outside and bring your butt down.

What will you experience during these exercises?

- **Excitation**. Because you imitate and emphasize the movements your body makes when it is getting close to climax, you could experience sexual excitation, tension in your sexual organs, heat and pleasure. Some women even reach orgasm during these exercises of breathing and motion!

- **Tingling sensation**. Breathing helps you circulate your sexual energy from your sexual organs throughout your body. You could feel it as a pleasant shiver or a tingling sensation in your palms, feet or mouth.

- **Relaxation and pleasure**. This is a way of becoming aware of your body, focusing on its reactions and needs and being in control, without feeling strained.

Can you use these techniques to achieve multiple orgasms? Yes, and here is how:

- After practicing for a few sessions and getting the motions and breathing integrated into your body's memory, you do not need to control them consciously. You will see that, during sex, they come naturally to prepare your body for orgasm and increase the intensity of your pleasure. Still, you can regain conscious control for a few minutes after an orgasm to in order to lead your body into the next one.

- Remember, a woman's sexual excitation follows an ascending curve, starting with stimulation and moving on to plateau, orgasm, another plateau, and then relaxation. If you catch the moment in the plateau after the first orgasm before the relaxation phase starts and use sexual stimulation again, you can restart the curve and have a second orgasm faster than the first.

- You can help your body prepare for this to happen by using the breathing and motion techniques. After the first orgasm, start breathing slowly, using breath retention and moving your pelvis. This will prepare your body for a second orgasm while allowing it to desensitize a little and be ready for additional touch.

- Duo Breathing

    1. Sit face to face with your partner, with legs crossed in the Lotus Position, with your knees touching your partner's knees. Keep your hands on each other's legs.

    2. Focus on your breathing. Do not make a special effort to synchronize your breathing; this will happen on its own. Inhale slowly, and then exhale slowly, at least 15 times.

What you need to remember is that these exercises will help you let go and enjoy sexual pleasure step by step. The longer you have been blocking your reactions, the longer it may take to unleash them, although this is not a fast rule; some women only need a little push to discover their inner sexual power and let it flow. The most difficult part is setting your mind free, so that it can reconnect to your body. When your mind, body, and spirit are connected, none of these are blocked any more, and you can experience a whole-body orgasm. If you love being in control, you may find this difficult; do not force yourself because relaxation never comes by force. Take things step by step: Today you let go a little, tomorrow some more, and then, before you know it, you will feel your mind, body, and spirit flow together as one.

Breathing Exercise for Deep Relaxation and Awakening

1. Lie down flat on your back, or sit or stand in any comfortable position as long as you are not bent at the waist or restricting your breathing in any way.

2. Select something beautiful to focus on, or close your eyes and mentally choose one of your favorite places. That could be a lush garden, a tranquil pool, a quiet sunset, or any visualization that feeds your senses gently in a relaxing way.

3. To begin, slowly breathe in as deeply as you can, and then exhale all the way. At first, you may need to use your hands to feel your ribs, then your diaphragm, then your belly, to make sure that they all expand. At the deepest point, you should feel expansion clear down to your belly and it should begin to rise.

4. You are in no hurry and should take breaths at a pleasant pace. If you feel any dizziness, breathe normally for a few breaths and then resume.

5. As you increase the number of deep breaths you can take in succession, focus on becoming increasingly relaxed with each breath, and the exercise will begin to seem rhythmic and effortless.

6. To complete the breathing exercise, exhale completely, making as much room as possible for the next cleansing breath.

Things to Know About Breathing

- If you are not used to deep breathing, you could experience dizziness, so it is best to lie down until you are accustomed to the exercise.

- The point of the breathing exercise is to breathe very deeply and gradually increase your ability to do this, so that it becomes a technique you can use whenever you need it.

- Also, as I often say, practice makes perfection. Practice a bit each day until you can do more and more of these breaths.

It is important when first practicing these exercises to consciously picture something beautiful and relaxing, so that your mind begins to associate this peaceful feeling with breathing deeply. The breathing will become automatic with practice and is to be used the moment negative or stressful thoughts intrude.

Distractions, even though you may be completely unaware of them, work against your body's ability to have an orgasm. Your mind can be wherever you wish it to be when you have an orgasm. But, for a woman, becoming stressed out will kill an orgasm.

Do not confuse this with having exciting fantasies, which is a totally different matter. It is quite common for a woman to use fantasies, like imagining her partner with another woman, being pursued sexually, or visualizing rougher sex than she actually likes in order to achieve orgasm. If these fantasies do not interfere, they are harmless. If you feel that a fantasy is negative for you, use the breathing to banish it.

The goal of breathing for relaxation during sex is twofold. You use it to remove unwanted or repetitive thoughts, like worrying about how you look, if you have any messages on your cell, or left the car unlocked. The moment one of these thoughts intrudes on your precious time for orgasm, immediately breathe deeply and picture your peaceful spot where all is beautiful and exactly as it should be.

At the end of the breathing exercise, exhale completely, making as much room as possible for the next cleansing breath. Practice a little each day until you can do more and more of these deep breaths.

Once you can maintain this breathing comfortably, you will begin to notice various tingling and warming sensations as tissues become enriched with blood and oxygen. This is like a foot waking up after it falls asleep and you begin moving it, but now all the tissues in your body awaken.

Oxygen always flows first to the vital organs like heart and brain, to sustain life. You need to keep breathing until the oxygen reaches all over, especially your genital area. As you slowly relax, your sexual organs are springing awake, and this means added pleasure for you.

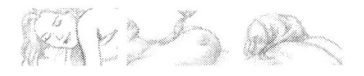

Invigorating Breathing Exercise for Awakening Orgasmic Pleasure

In order to experience sensual pleasure and achieve orgasm, it is essential to learn to be present in your body in order to experience sensations, as well as to be free of anxiety and quiet in your mind.

An exercise you can practice to begin to quiet the mind and awaken the body is the invigorating breathing exercise. This will help your body become more aware of the stimuli it is receiving. Also, by counting, your mind will focus only on the here and now, relaxing and allowing you to be fully present in the experience you are having.

1. Exhale fully and slowly while counting from 10 down to 1.
2. Slowly inhale again counting back from 10 to 1. Remember to focus on your breathing and counting.
3. Hold your breath for the same count: 10 to 1
4. Slowly release the breath from 10 to 1.

5. Practice daily, starting with 3 breaths and increasing by one breath each day.

6. Allow this breathing to be a training process. If your body feels as though you have had enough, stop. Listen inwardly with compassion.

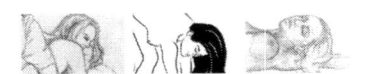

Motivational Moment

You now have three powerful breathing techniques that you will return to again and again to remain fully in each present moment with your pleasure spots energized and nourished from head to toe, ready to respond to the ecstasy that awaits you. You may use the mantra suggested or create your own to remind you to breathe.

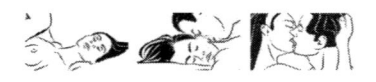

Note about the Tantric Breath of Love

This chapter emphasizes my belief in using specific breathing techniques at the right moments to enhance every aspect of female sexual pleasure and allow the woman to experience amazing and multiple orgasms. The different breathing exercises, while easy, are described in detail to allow you to both practice them often and use them correctly as needed.

Fill out the following chart to keep the record of the result of your exercises:

1. Which breathing exercise did you do this week: Nirvana dance, Deep Relaxation and Awakening, Orgasmic Pleasure, Duo Breathing?

2. What change do you want to see in yourself spiritually and sexually?

3. How do you feel about your own sexuality now you have done these exercises?

4. From 1 to 10, rate how these exercises improve the quality of your orgasms(s).

	1	2	3	4
Week 1				
Week 2				
Week 3				
Week 4				
Week 5				
Week 6				
Week 7				
Week 8				

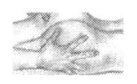

CHAPTER 3

Tantric Massage

What is Tantric Massage?

As I sit here and reflect on Zarah, everything comes back to me in waves. This woman was so full of passion and life. She was one of those people that no matter how dark the world around her got, she remained optimistic and bright.

Clicking on the e-mail from Zarah, I scanned the information she had provided: "I am in my mid-thirties, a beautiful blonde with long, shining locks. Your massage sounds delightful! I'm thinking about giving it a try; I really need some release."

"I live in Malibu in a little beachside condo; you know the kind: palm trees in the front yard with Spanish moss growing from their trunks, and the ocean in the backyard, the waves. The sea is usually so calming, but not for me anymore."

"So much has happened in the last year. I'm so stressed. The economy is flat lining, every dollar is harder to earn and doesn't go quite as far. I feel beaten. I could really use a massage that will help shift my state. Please let me know if you would be interested in working on me."

There was an interest in massage in Zarah's note, which I enjoyed seeing, because Tantric massage is about the awakening and fulfillment *of fantasy for the woman. I wrote back and explained to Zarah that Tantric massage is an intimate way of connecting on a spiritual level via the contact of flesh.*

"I use warm oil to give body a slow, gentle massage; this relaxes each and every one of your muscles," I told her. "As your body relaxes, your mind and spirit will be in a free-meditative state and open to me. We create a cleansing spiritual bond with rhythmic breathing, full relaxation, and the power of flesh upon flesh."

"Of course, we must build rapport and strengthen trust in one another. In order for us to get to this point, it is important to spend time talking and getting to know each other first."

I do Tantric massage to bring men and women close to each other. Once you learn the secrets of Tantra, you will feel secure in your sexuality, and men will adore you. If we can bring women and men closer to each other, we will have peace in this world.

I believe that when we bring men and women closer to each other, women will influence men, and we will have fewer wars. Yes! The power of the feminine will temper that of the masculine—softening and strengthening men at the same time—and this will change the world.

Addressing Zarah once again, I wrote, "Once a woman reaches the level of freedom, intensity and pleasure available through Tantra, she will have a smile on her face forever. Through massage, I make each woman feel like a woman, and she will know her inner feminine power."

Zarah replied, "I feel very reassured, and of course I would very much like to try the massage! I have read about Tantra and Taoist sexual yoga, but never had a partner or masseur who was trained in it. I will be waiting for you. . . ."

Tantric massage is an old form of holistic massage that addresses the mind, body, and soul. (*see drawing: Tantric massage is an old form of holistic massage that addresses the mind, body, and soul.*) Associated with sensuality, unity, and getting in touch with your partner's body, Tantra has become an art for the healing of both body and mind. The word *Tantra* means "to extend knowledge," and that is exactly what Tantric massage does: It extends your perceptions, your sensuality, and your mind.

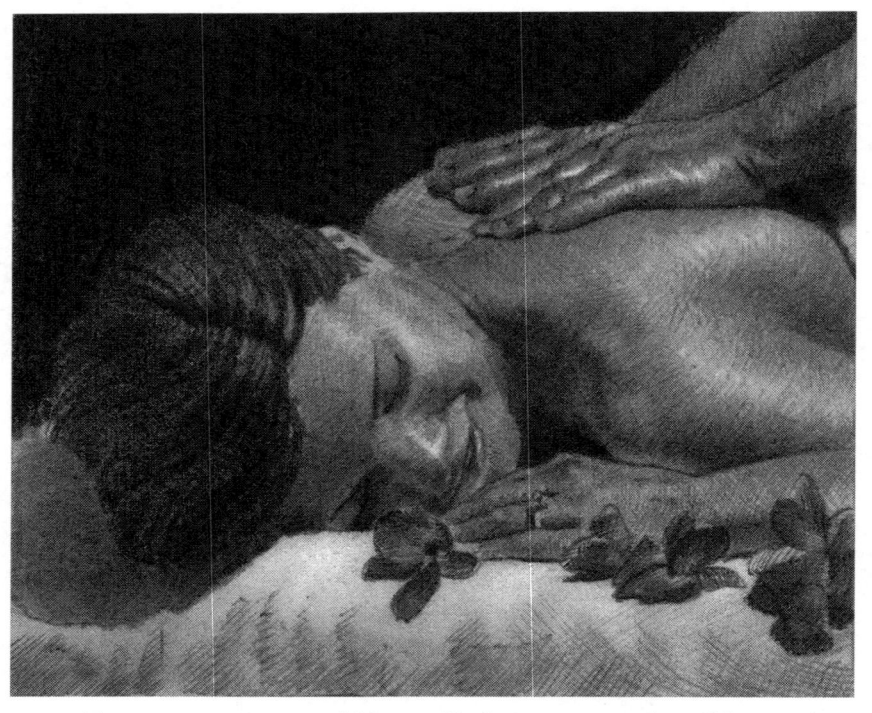

Tantric massage is an old form of holistic massage that addresses the mind, body, and soul

Although there is much to learn about Tantra and Tantric massage, there are no rules and nothing to stop you from getting started with your partner (or on your own) right away. This is a freestyle massage, as long as it is gentle. Tantra is a journey, and with your body, imagination and open mind, you have the most important tools you will need right at hand.

Some women are more sensitive to massage than others, they become instinctively aroused when you begin to massage while other women will take more time and work. Sensuality, in the same way as sexuality (which is our ability to have an orgasm), depends of our mental blocks caused by emotional tension. As human beings we are all originally extremely sensual and sexual, but the conditions and the experience of our life leave us in difference state of sensitivity. Tantra is here to help you to open up and enjoy that vast amount of pleasure that your body has to offer.

Hint for a Male Lover

Often, men are more prone to do things than to feel them and just follow the flow. A man's nature is to expect something when he gives; the nature of a woman is to be able to receive without expectation. The more a man can take the initiative to intuit what pleases his partner or ask her what pleases her, the more she will feel that she has been heard, seen, and understood. Many women also want to give Tantric massage to a partner, and a woman should approach this gift that she will give with the same spirit of love, passion, and sharing. The idea is to set up an environment within which both of you can explore the heights of your sensuality and sexuality—an activity that can greatly enhance the emotional intimacy between you.

Setting the Atmosphere

Welcome to a delicious journey of endless awakenings. Take the time and care to prepare your setting, so that you can allow your adventure to unfold. You will need to gather information about your likes and dislikes, and find the perfect items to entice, tease, and let your physical and emotional excitement progress in the fashion that is right for you. Allowing yourself enough time to get to know your emotional and physical body can lead to a heightened vulnerability. This openness may with time take you to new heights of intensity.

Space and Time

In setting the stage for Tantric massage, the physical space and timing are two of the most important aspects of this experience. It is vital that the location you choose for this exploration is secure, private, and free of any distractions as well as time constraints. The goal is to eliminate any external pressures that could raise anxiety and have negative effect on your own and your partner's psychological state. The goal is to create an environment that honors your vulnerability and facilitates awareness and a focus on the pleasures, thereby enabling your body to respond without interference from anxiety, guilt, or limiting thoughts.

Preparation

Preparing for Tantric massage alone can begin to arouse a woman's senses. Listen to your internal self to find out what seduces your senses. What do you consider sensual? What do you consider visually beautiful? What types of touch causes the slightest bit of arousal? What kind of sounds create tingling in your breast and groin?

The process of gathering objects and tools that speak to and enhance your unique sensuality will beautifully set the stage for your massage. The following are some tantalizing ideas that address the senses, but remember that this is your experience, your journey:

Visual Voyage

Pastel fresh flowers, burning candles in soft colors, satin or velvet sheets in your favorite color are all items that speak to the visual side of your sensual nature. To arouse your sensual and sexual urges further, you may choose to use these or other items to dramatize or act out a forbidden desire. You may also find reading an erotic novel or watching a video of a guilty pleasure or fantasy visually stimulating.

Radiant Fragrances

Use fragrance in the form of scented candles, scented massage oils, incense, a scented oil lamp, or of course scented flowers to awaken another part of your sensuality through the sense of smell. Tip for men: Men's colognes or incense can be too strong for some women; get to know the types of scents that your woman enjoys.

Soothing Sounds

Sound expresses feelings and sensuality and seduces the soul. Sound that loosely envelops and touches you deeply will enhance your Tantric massage experience. Some suggestions include quiet music that you love, sounds of the ocean, or music with meditative, hypnotic rhythms.

Tantalizing Tastes

Taste is an intricate part of sensual message. Tasting is orally stimulating and excites the senses through both aroma and flavor. Some flavorful hints include chocolate-dipped strawberries with long stems, whipped cream, champagne, and chocolate or vanilla fondue.

In addition to their fascinating scents and flavors, some foods actually have aphrodisiac effects that could help you relax and get in the mood. Some of the ones that work best for women:

Chocolate: No wonder so many women are crazy about chocolate. Dark chocolate contains phenyl ethylamine, a chemical that assists in the release of serotonin, which is also sometimes called "the hormone of happiness." Serotonin is also released while exercising or having sex and when you are in love.

Vanilla: The scent of vanilla helps you become more relaxed and is a great mood enhancer. Drink a vanilla tea or have it in your dessert in order to forget your daily problems and focus on the connection between you and your partner.

Almonds: In ancient writings, almonds were considered to improve fertility and sexual desire in women. Try eating some almond paste (marzipan) as a late-night treat and see its sweet effects in the bedroom.

And here are some aphrodisiac foods for men:

Ginger: The substance that gives the ginger its spiciness is the same one that improves blood circulation in your whole body, including your sexual organs. Add a little to whatever you are having for dinner, in order to spice things up in the bedroom as well as on your plate.

Honey: The food of bees is rich in vitamin B, and this helps with the production of sex hormones. In other words, honey puts you in the mood. The same applies to other bee products such as pollen.

Bananas: This popular fruit contains bromelain, an enzyme that increases male libido. Also, its phallic shape makes it the perfect choice for a sensual game during foreplay, when your partner could slowly eat a banana in front of you.

If you share these foods, the two of you will each experience relaxation, increased sexual appetite, and intense orgasms:

Avocado: The vitamin B contained in avocado increases male hormone production, and its potassium regulates a woman's thyroid, which controls the receptivity of the body to the production of hormones.

Oysters: The amino acids in oysters increase the production of sex hormones, and the zinc they contain helps with the production of testosterone, the male hormone responsible for the libido in both sexes.

Wine: Any kind of alcohol, in small quantities, helps partners to relax and become more focused on their bodies. But wine has many properties, including its color, scent, and flavor, that enhance and open the senses, like a glass of champagne. The tannin contained in grapes also boosts fertility, in both men and women. I have also noticed women tend to request Tantric massage far more often during the fertile phase than at any other time of the month! (see drawing: *But wine has many properties, including its color, scent, and flavor, that enhance and open the senses, like a glass of champagne*)

Weed: If you live in California or somewhere in the world where weed, cannabis, is authorized or medically prescribed, I would suggest to try it, as it might help you to enjoy your sexual pleasure. Some women reported to me that they achieved multiple orgasms when they were high. Ancient Tantrists noticed and agreed that people who enjoy sex also enjoy marijuana. Cannabis has been used in India for over 3000 years as the ultimate aphrodisiac that conquers impotence and frigidity.

Garlic: Although the smell of garlic is not the most beautiful scent in the world, both of you should try eating it for better sex. Garlic contains allicin, which increases the blood flow to the sexual organs, including the penis and clitoris, making women more sensitive to touch and helping men to keep an erection for longer.

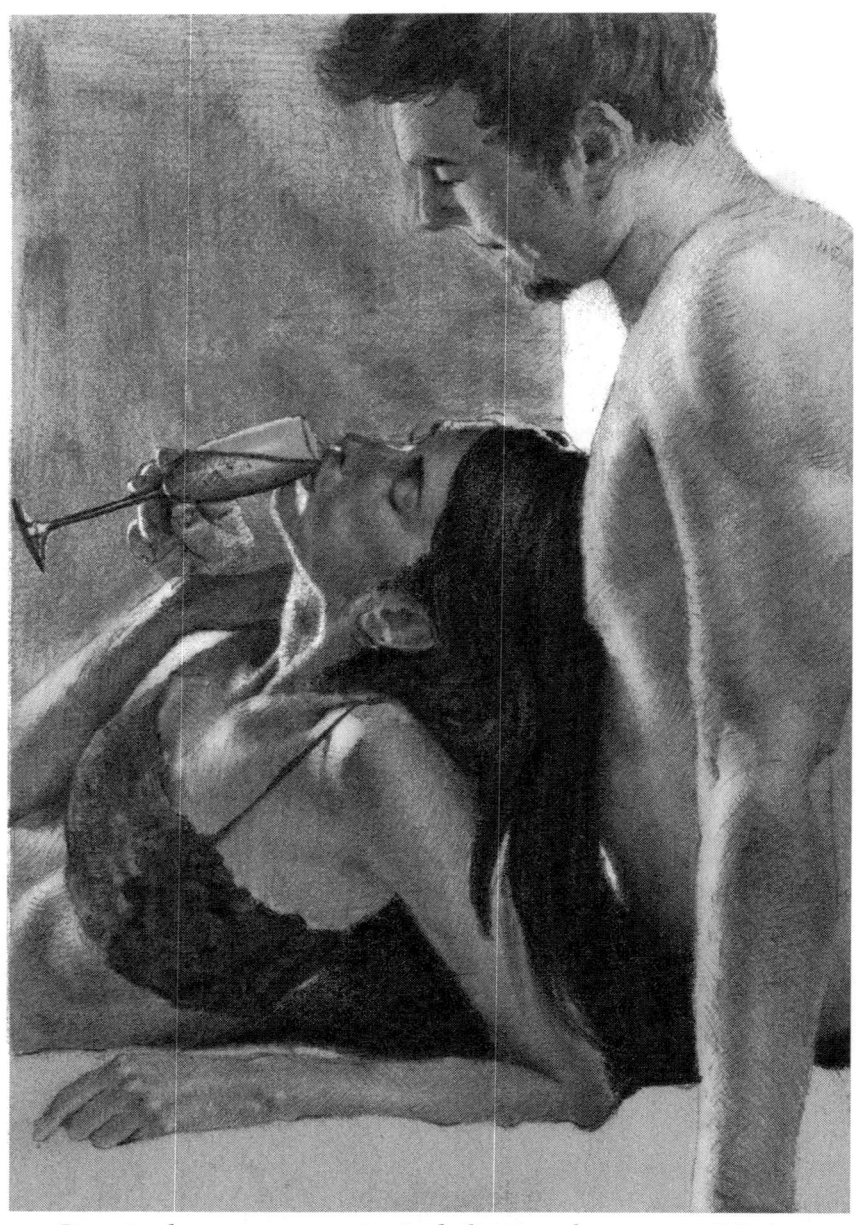

But wine has many properties, including its color, scent, and flavor, that enhance and open the senses, like a glass of champagne

Some of these foods are best eaten over long-term periods, as new habits, to ensure their aphrodisiac effects in your sensual life. However, sharing some strawberries dipped in dark chocolate sauce or licking honey from your partner's body, for instance, could be an interesting prelude to or stimulating part of our massage experience. Besides the erotic show that licking offers your lover, there is also a personal benefit: In the *Kama Sutra*, it is said that enjoying a mix of honey and nutmeg will heighten orgasm for both partners. So . . . have fun, and *bon appétit!*

Tactile Delight

The tactile sense encompasses the body's physical perceptions of pressure, temperature, and pain and pleasure from touch, both internally and externally — in other words, all of the physical experiences of one body surface coming into contact with that of another body or objects. The range of possible sensual experience through touch is broad. Some possibilities for your massage include a warm temperature; a comfortable bed or sofa; a thick comfortable rug; velvet, silk, or satin sheets and pillow cases; comfortable pillows; thick, soft towels; robe and slippers; heated body butter or massage oil; all types of vibrators, butt plugs, and dildos.

Setting the Stage

Once you have chosen the space and the specific objects of seduction, it is time to set your stage. The following are only some ideas for consideration. Take your time and set up your massage space just for you. This sacred area will come together solely for the exploration of your pleasure. Be sure to notice any tinges of excitement or sexual arousal as you prepare your sanctuary. Keep handy all the materials you will need for an erotic massage: feathers, scent, oil, sexual enhancers, candles, vibrator, blindfold, scarf, glass of wine or champagne, and towels in different sizes. Your Goddess will appreciate how you will wash her body in the most intimate way once the massage is over.

Once your massage space is ready and waiting, it may be more dramatic and delicious to wait an hour or two before starting your massage. This will enable you to take in the full impression of your creation and allow the setting to envelop you.

You may wish to take a ceremonial bath in preparation for your massage and to rest after all of your exertions. When, after an hour or so, you enter your scared space, allow yourself to be awestruck by all of your sensual perceptions. Allow yourself to be drawn to whatever you feel is comfortable and begin to explore.

When you perform a Tantric massage, let yourself explore and caress your partner's whole body. In Tantra, all parts of the body are treated with equal care, and there is no shame or revulsion toward some body parts. All parts of the body are beautiful (and possibly erogenous!), so explore them all.

Here are some tips for a successful and satisfying Tantric massage:

Every Tantric massage starts with the energy connection between your eyes and those of your partner. Gaze at your partner, and let your eyes spark as you think of her as the Goddess of sensuality. Your partner needs to be appreciated and adored the way she is, with every wrinkle, scar, or grey hair. You are the God of virility, and your job is to pleasure her. When her inner energy is awakened, she will radiate love and sexuality, independently of her age or physical appearance. She will feel beautiful through your eyes, and so she will become beautiful.

Email received *"Dear Jean-Claude My reasons for contacting you are many.*

The first one is that my sexual experiences for the past three years (with the same man) have been superficially and intense. Sometimes I have had orgasms..most times not. He thought that intensity was all that was needed, when what was really needed was a relaxed passion that catered to every part of my body; which ultimately would cause the intensity. He was rarely a part of the experience. Instead his goal was to make me cum, not to make me feel fantastic.

With that said, I'm not seeing him anymore and I want to experience sensuality like I've never experienced before. I feel and think that I need to avail myself to this as a way of taking care of me. I've always wanted sensuality to rise to a spiritual level; where the point is for both parties to please beyond belief.

Also, I want to learn about my body. I've read what you've sent and I would like to be aware of myself sexually; how I can be affected and how I can affect.

Most men aim for the end result and are not available for the journey; which leaves most women not getting our needs met.

So, yes, I am e-mailing because I want to learn about sensuality; how to give it and how to accept it.

Can you teach me? If so, when?" Erica G.

Here are some suggestion and advice on how to get started with Tantric massages:

- For a wonderful Tantric massage, use scented oil. Choose a natural herbal massage oil made from organic plants. Heat it a little before the massage, so it will feel pleasant, not cold. Never apply the oil directly to your partner's body; instead, pour a little oil onto your hands, rub them together, and then start the massage. Re-apply the oil whenever necessary. Remember, your hands should slide easily on your partner's body, but they should not drip with oil. That would be too oily!

- Speak to your partner when massaging her, and choose your words carefully, to make this experience completely arousing. The connection and trust between the two of you (the giver of the massage and the receiver) are the most important ingredients in Tantric massage.

- Start with massage of the backside, as your Goddess will feel less vulnerable. Ask your woman to lie on the bed face down, with her arms alongside her body and her legs spread a little. It is better to massage from a less sensitive area and move on to more sensitive areas later. The spinal area is usually less sensitive than other spots, so this is a good place to start. The most sensitive areas of the backside are the feet, hips, lower back, neck, lobe of the ear, and buttocks, and they should be massaged later on. The massage should start with slow motions and move on to become more intense. After you finish massaging her shoulder butt and head, your partner can turn over, allowing you to massage her front, too, starting from the head and moving to the toes. (*see drawing: After you finish massaging her shoulder, butt and head*)

- Some of the advantages of Tantric massage, for both women and men, are:

For a woman, Tantric massage will improve your receptivity to touch, make you more aware of your body's needs, increase your femininity, and allow you to discover your inner Goddess. The practice of Tantric massage can help you address emotional and sexual blockages due to experiences that you may have had in the past. Just close your eyes during the massage, and visualize everything that you want from life at this moment. Maybe you want more confidence, or love, or more powerful orgasms; just relax and imagine you already have them. Through Tantric massage you will awaken a powerful orgasmic energy that will allow you to have better and multiple orgasms, experience orgasmic bliss, and also make your wishes come true.

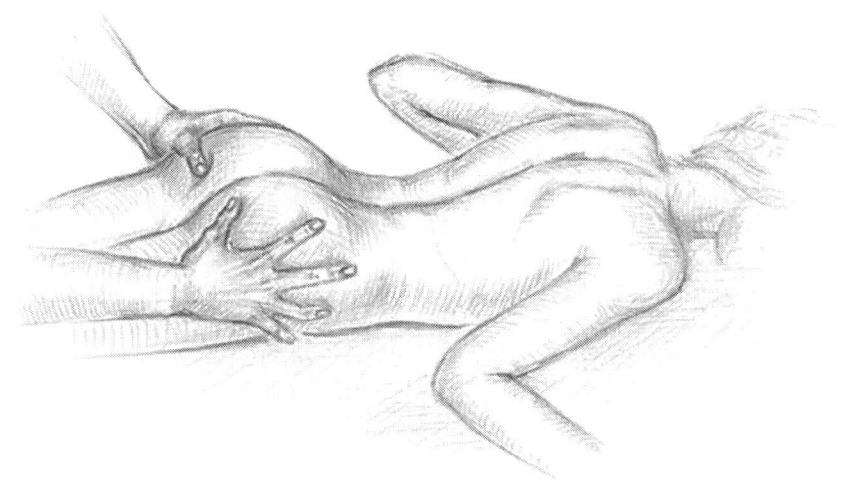

After you finish massaging her shoulder butt and head

- For men, the Tantric massage they perform on a partner will help them open sexually and be more receptive to the woman's suggestions and needs. The Tantric massage you receive from your Goddess partner will allow you to create a powerful connection between the two of you and to better control your sexual energy and ejaculation.

Because of the complexity of its purpose—the unity of body, mind and spirit—Tantric massage includes a variety of techniques that are explained below. There is no strict pattern in Tantric massage. You can use your hands, your mouth, your hair, a feather or any object that causes a pleasant sensation on or in the Goddess's body. Take time to try all of them. Each has its own special flavor, and every woman has her favorite.

Massage with a Feather

This Tantric massage technique consists of very soft touches using only a feather. Try different types of feathers: ostrich, peacock, or eagle, in order to produce different sensations. The direction of the massage should be from feet to vulva and then from head to vulva, leaving the most sensitive and sexual part for the end. When performing a feather massage on your Goddess's body: (*see drawing: This Tantric massage technique consists of very soft touches using only a feather*)

- Start with her feet and move up. If she is ticklish, use a drop of massage oil, preferably something minty, and apply it to her feet with your hands; the tingly oil will desensitize her feet at first, and then intensify the sensations. Caress her feet with the feather, touching them softly or patting them gently. Gently draw the feather through her toes, and use it to explore every inch of her feet, from her heels to the tips of her toes and from her toenails up to her ankles.

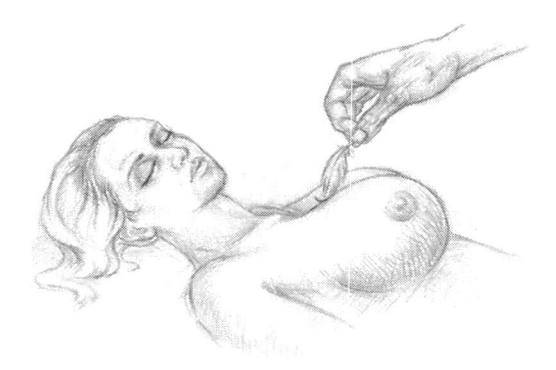

This Tantric massage technique consists of very soft touches using only a feather

- After applying a little oil on her back, use the feather to massage your Goddess's back. Let the feather slide along the spine to the small of her back and back up. Caress your Goddess's ears, neck and face with the softness of the feather until her every pore is aroused. Do not neglect the breasts or her arms. Play with her nipples, caressing them with soft touches, and outline her breasts with gentle touches of the feather. Move down the abdomen, to the pubic area, before giving special attention to the yoni (vulva).

- The softness touché of the feather will help to spread her legs, so that you have access to her inner thighs and yoni. Use the feather to gently tap her labia, and caress the perinea. Move from the inner thigh to her vulva and then back, surprising her with your motions. Her labia will open gently, and caress her clitoris with the feather, using circular motions and up-and-down motions, moving from her clitoris to her vagina.

Oral Massage

When it comes to oral massage, one of women's favorites, you only use your lips and tongue to touch your partner's whole body. Massaging your partner with your tongue offers both you and your Goddess a sensual, delicious experience. Here are a few suggestions for oral massage of your partner's body:

- Use strokes and touches of different intensities. This will allow your partner to experience a wide variety of sensations. Do not be afraid to lick and suck. Use your tongue and lips to discover your partner's erogenous areas, some of which she may not even know she has.

- Ask your partner to keep her eyes closed, and lick her eyelids. Move the tip of your tongue on her cheeks, upper lip and ears. Explore her ear lobes with your mouth, suck them, and lick the outlines of her ears. This is a very sensitive area for many women, so pay attention to your partner's reactions. Lick her neck and the back of her neck, and then slide your tongue along her spine.

- Lick or gently bite her buttocks, and then move your tongue down her leg, giving special attention to the backs of her knees. Kiss her legs up and down, then take time to fondle her feet. Some of the most erogenous areas a woman have are her feet and toes. Suck every toe, slide your tongue through her toes, and then gently lick her heels and ankles. It will drive her crazy. Some women may even have an orgasm during a Tantric foot massage.

Massage with the Tips of the Fingers

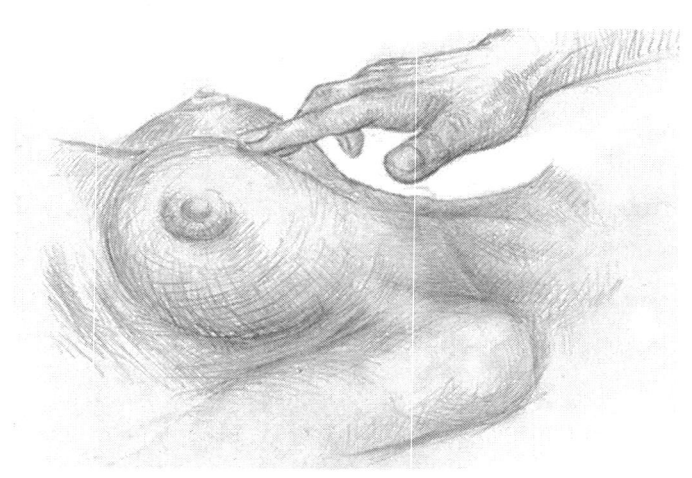

You can write sexy messages on your partner's skin and let her guess what you wrote

This is a special Tantric massage technique that provides a wide variety of sensations to your partner using only the tips of your fingers. You can use your fingers to gently touch her skin or to apply a little pressure in specific areas and transform this experience into a mind-blowing, sensual massage.

- Use a drop of oil on your fingers, to make your touches more pleasant and arousing. Surprise is the key element in this technique. Use both soft touches and intense ones, and draw soft circles or imitate the rain drops on your partner's skin. Be playful. You can write sexy messages on your partner's skin and let her guess what you wrote. (*see drawing: You can write sexy messages on your partner's skin and let her guess what you wrote*)

- Start with the face, gently outlining your partner's eyebrows, nose, cheeks, and lips. Apply a little tap at the end of the eyebrows, on the cheekbones, and above the upper lip. Some energy nodes are stimulated by gentle tapping, allowing energy to flow freely through your partner's body.

- Massage your partner's shoulders, arms, hands, breasts, abdomen, and legs. Linger on your partner's buttocks and vulva. Remember that the purpose of the massage is to arouse the skin and awaken energy. (*see drawing: Massage your partner's hands*)

Breast Massage

Most women usually feel their partner do not pay enough attention to their breast or they are too rough. One of women's most important sexual receptors, the breasts, can be stimulated by hand, by mouth, or with different objects, a silk scarf, for example. There is a strong connection between the breasts and the clitoris; the stimulation of one also produces excitation in the other. By stimulating the nipples, oxytocin is liberated into the brain. Oxytocin, also known as the "love hormone," will give your Goddess a higher level of pleasure and prepare her body for orgasm. The most receptive women may even experience orgasm from breast stimulation only! So, take time to please your partner by exploring her breasts through Tantric massage. (*see drawing: Take time to please your partner by exploring her breasts through Tantric massage*)

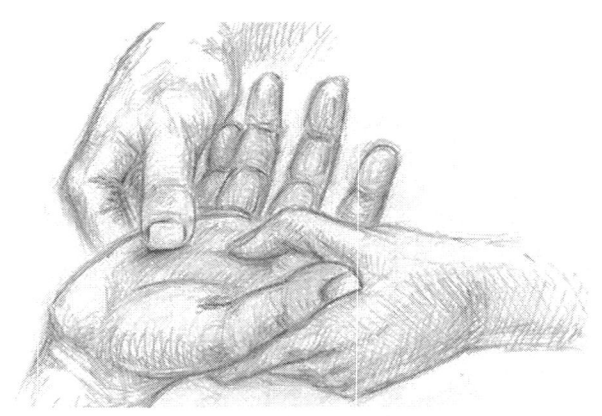

Massage your partner's hands

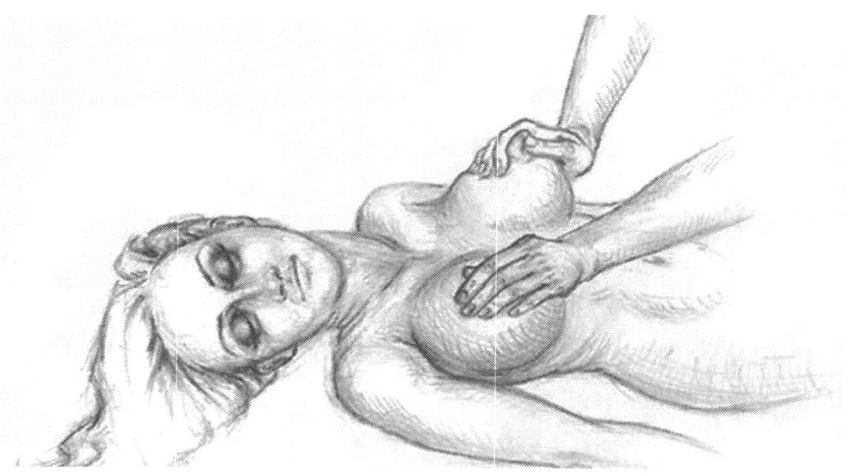

Take time to please your partner by exploring her breasts through Tantric massage

- Use a little massage oil to prepare the breasts for massage. Start by caressing the breasts first, with the tips of your fingers; first use soft touches, and then add more pressure. Knead the breasts gently, always paying attention to your partner's reaction. See if she likes the pressure or rhythm that you are using.

- Do not begin to touch your Goddess by touching her nipples. It is important to touch that very sensitive part of her body only once she is already aroused. When her nipple is erect, touch it delicately, by describing circles around the areola, then squeeze the nipple between your fingers. Gently pull it away than release it. Now you might also massage the breast and the nipple with your lips and tongue. Take the nipple in your mouth, suck it gently, and then release it. If you blow some air on the nipple while it is wet and erect, this will make your partner moan with pleasure. Adapt your touches according to your partner's feedback: If she moans, moves her hips, or bites her lips with pleasure, then you are doing it right.

- Next, move your nose around her nipples, smell her nipples, and give a long lick all over her erected breast.

- Then slowly take the whole breast in your mouth, take in as much as you can. Same as you wish she does for your penis. Gently use your teeth against her breast and keep her nipple deep in your mouth as long as you can.

Back, Hip and Spine Massage

Massaging the back, hips, and spine relieves stress and pressure and also stimulates sensuality by opening the Svadhisthana chakra at the lower end of the spine. Always use massage oil to prepare her skin for your touches, and use both large and more concentrated touches.

Use some warm oil to prepare your hands and your partner's back for the sensual touches that are to follow. Start with the top of the spine, and apply a little pressure while you let your thumb slide down to the place where the buttocks meet. Blow over her spine, retracing the touches of your hands. You can also use your tongue to wet her skin, adding sensation to the spine massage. Remember, the purpose of Tantric massage is to relax and stimulate the skin, not to massage the muscles, so use soft, sensual touches, not deep ones.

- Gently draw lines with your fingers on your partner's back and spine. Do not forget about the shoulders, because a lot of negative energy accumulates in the shoulders. With your oiled hands, stimulate your partner's shoulders and upper back. Release the negative energy using broad circular motions. When stimulating her shoulders, apply light pressure with your hands stacked one on top of the other, and continue the massage that way.

- When you reach the hips, use your open palms to massage your partner with circular motions. This is a very sensual massage that stimulates the second chakra, responsible for sexuality and sensuality. Be generous to your partner, and you will feel her blossom under your hands like the Goddess that she is. (*see drawing: When you reach the hips, use your open palms to massage your partner with circular motions*)

Legs, Inner Thigh and Foot Massage

When massaging these lower parts of the body, always start with the feet and then work your way up the leg. Use warm massage oil and go easy, especially on the feet; some women have very sensitive feet and are ticklish. Adapt your touches' strength and rhythm according to your partner's wishes. Repeat every move three to four times, so that her skin has time to enjoy them and to allow her energy to arise.

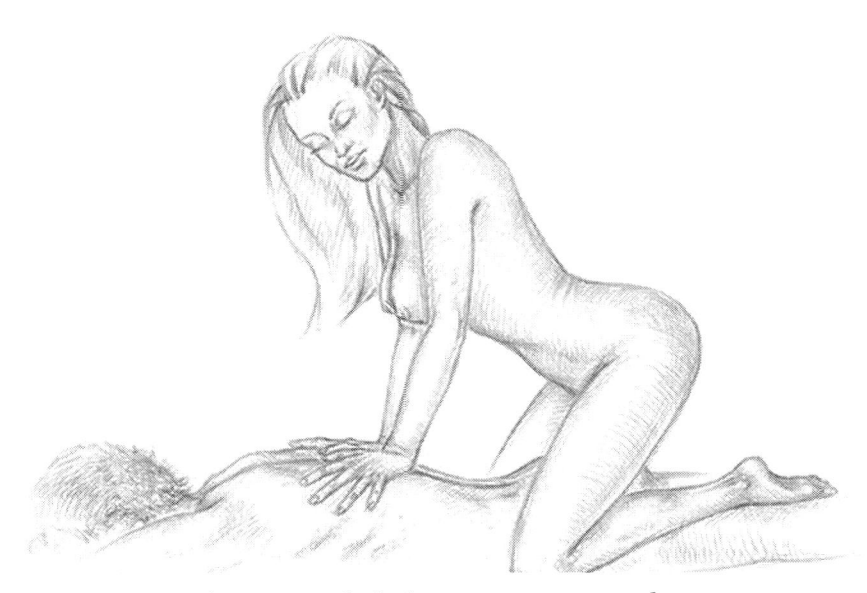

When you reach the hips, use your open palms to massage your partner with circular motions

- Often women who have manicured feet are more sensitive in that area. Use both of your hands, one on top of the foot and one underneath. With her foot enclosed like a delicate flower, use your thumbs to slide up and down along the soles of her feet, and then in circular motions. Feet are very erogenous areas, and some women may experience orgasm through oral and hand massage of the feet. Caress her toes with your mouth, lick them, and suck them one by one. The sensations your partner will experience will bring her closer to heaven.

- When moving up your partner's legs, use your fingers and your fingertips to stimulate the skin, especially around the knees and the outer thighs. Around the kneecap, work in circular

- It is better if your partner lies on her stomach as you gently massage her inner thighs. Women are more sensitive to the touches that come from the rear. Stroke your partner's inner thigh gently, from the knee to the groin. You can also use your knuckles and the tips of your fingers to imitate the rain falling on her thighs.

Anal Massage

Tantric massage of the anal area should be given with care and tenderness. This is not an area to be stimulated at the beginning of a Tantric massage session but can be prepared for gently by helping your partner to relax during the massage of her whole body.

- Delicately ask your Goddess to lie on her stomach with a pillow under her belly. Another position for this technique would be for her to lie on her back, with a pillow under her hips, legs apart, and knees bent.

- Start by massaging your partner's hips and buttocks, and then gently slide between the buttocks. Use some water-based lubricant, because massage oil could harm this sensitive area.

motions using both of your hands. Use both hands to glide up to the groin, with one hand behind the other. Do this slowly, without changing your rhythm.

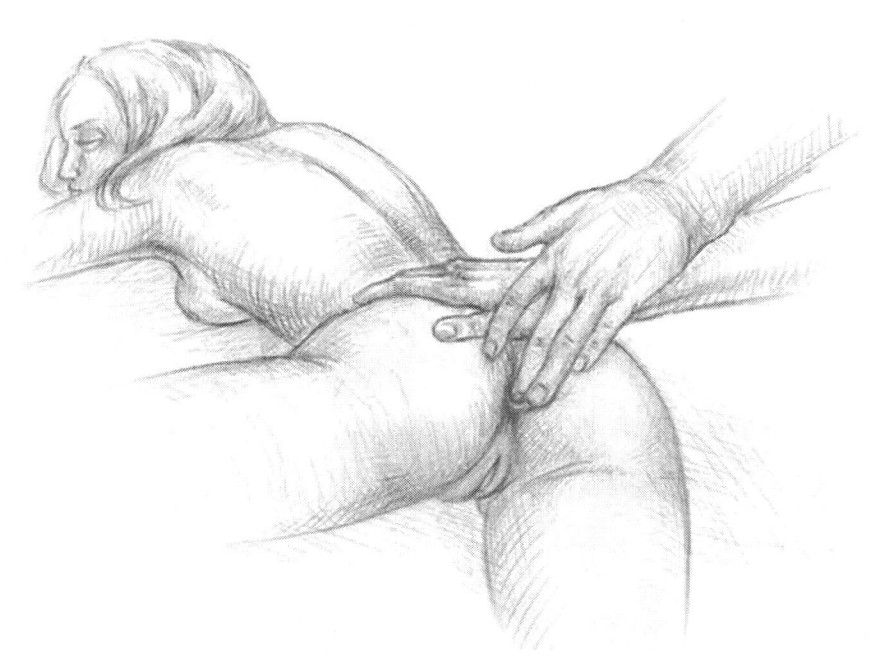

With one hand, spread the buttocks, and with the other, stimulate the anus

- Warm the lubricant in your hands before applying it. Use up and down motions to stimulate the anus. With one hand, spread the buttocks, and with the other, stimulate the anus. You can also use your tongue to massage the rosebud (anus) and help her relax her muscles. (*see drawing: With one hand, spread the buttocks, and with the other, stimulate the anus*)

- After a while, if your partner feels comfortable and aroused, add more lubricant, and use your finger to penetrate your partner anally. At first use your pinky, and slowly stroke the walls of the anus. Use an in-and-out motion, as well as circular ones. As your partner becomes more aroused, you can add another finger or two. Do not forget about the lubricant, as the anal channel does not have natural lubrication like the vagina. (*see drawing: Use your finger to penetrate your partner anally.*)

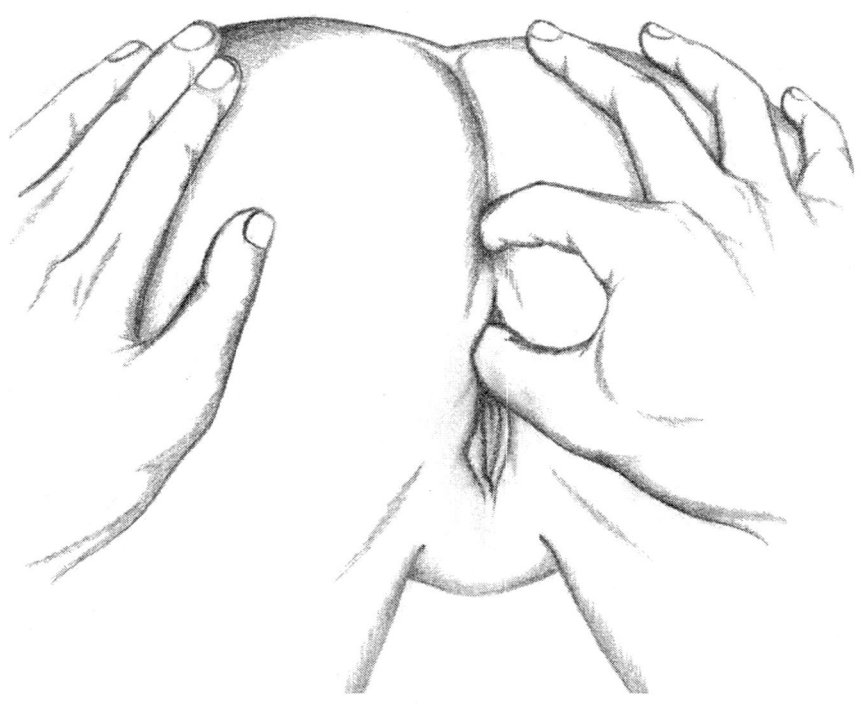

Use your finger to penetrate your partner anally

- For a more complete experience, you can add stimulation of the vagina and the clitoris at the same time. This triple stimulation can lead to an explosive orgasm and even to ejaculation from the "Goddess's fountain" as you simultaneously massage her G-spot through the thin wall of the anus and through the vagina. It is call the bracket (*see drawing: For a more complete experience, you can add stimulation of the vagina and the clitoris at the same time*)

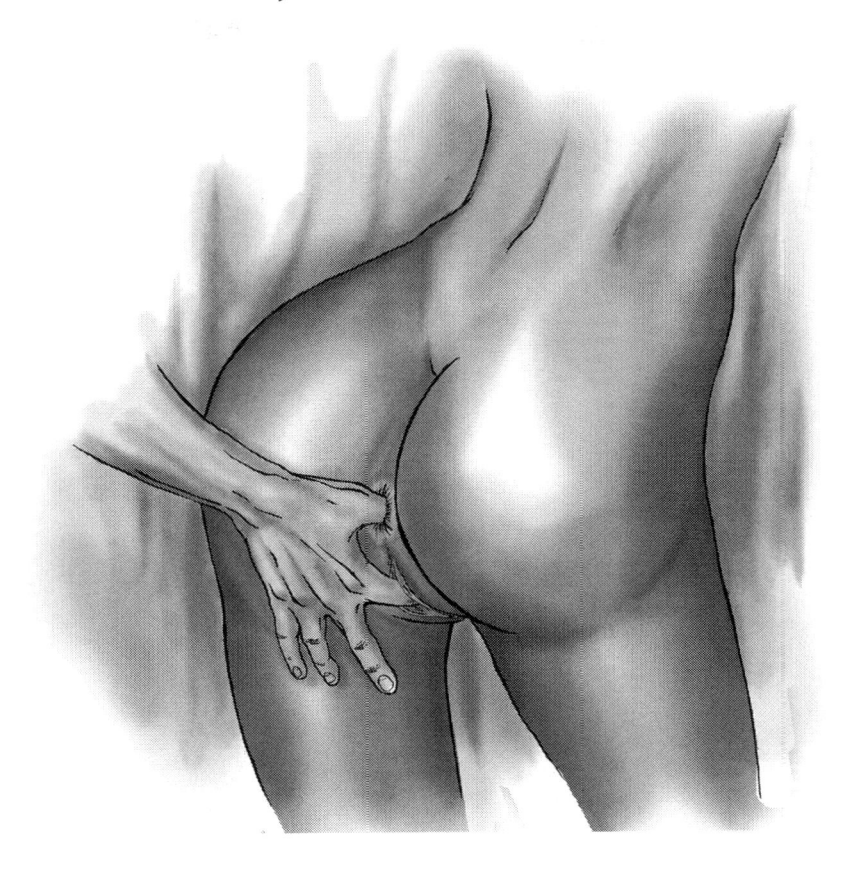

For a more complete experience, you can add stimulation of the vagina and the clitoris at the same time

If your woman does not ejaculate during your first trials of this technique during massage, do not give up or feel too disappointed. Mastering the technique for G-spot massage and getting in touch with those sensations will almost certainly take time for you both. Read Chapter 7 and Chapter 8 in this book. Practice vaginal stimulation of the G-spot once a week to see results very soon.

Head and Neck Massage

Because it is usually covered with hair, the skin of the head is rarely touched directly, and this is why it is more sensitive during massages. For your Goddess's head massage, do not massage only with your fingers. You can massage her face, lips, and neck, along with the rest of her head. Most women love head massage, and they will appreciate a lover who pays attention to this area of the body.

- For face massage, your motions should follow the lines of her face: horizontal on the forehead and cheekbones, vertical on the nose, and circular on the temples. Use the tips of your fingers to massage her lips and trace their outline. Also massage her with your lips, hair, and nose. Get close to her skin, and let her feel your deep breathing as you massage.

- Do not neglect her ears, a very erogenous area. Squeeze her earlobes between your fingers, and gently trace their outlines with the tip of a finger, following their curves. Massage the lobes with your tongue, suck on them gently. Be playful and sensual.

- For her neck, use a little massage oil, and massage both the back and front of the neck. The nape should be massaged using your whole hand; place your hand with open palm on one side of the nape, drape your fingers across her neck, and then slowly pull your fingers across the nape until your palm closes. Add a little pressure, but not so much that it is painful. Massage her neck with your tongue, and then blow warm air across it. It will surely arouse her! (*see drawing: The nape should be massaged using your whole hand; place your hand with open palm on one side of the nape*)

Arm and Hand Massage

In our palms are the two chakras that connect us to other people and help us establish a level of intimacy in our relationships. For this reason, the palms should always be treated with care and gifted with a lot of love and tenderness. When performing a Tantric massage, you should definitely give special attention to your partner's arms and hands.

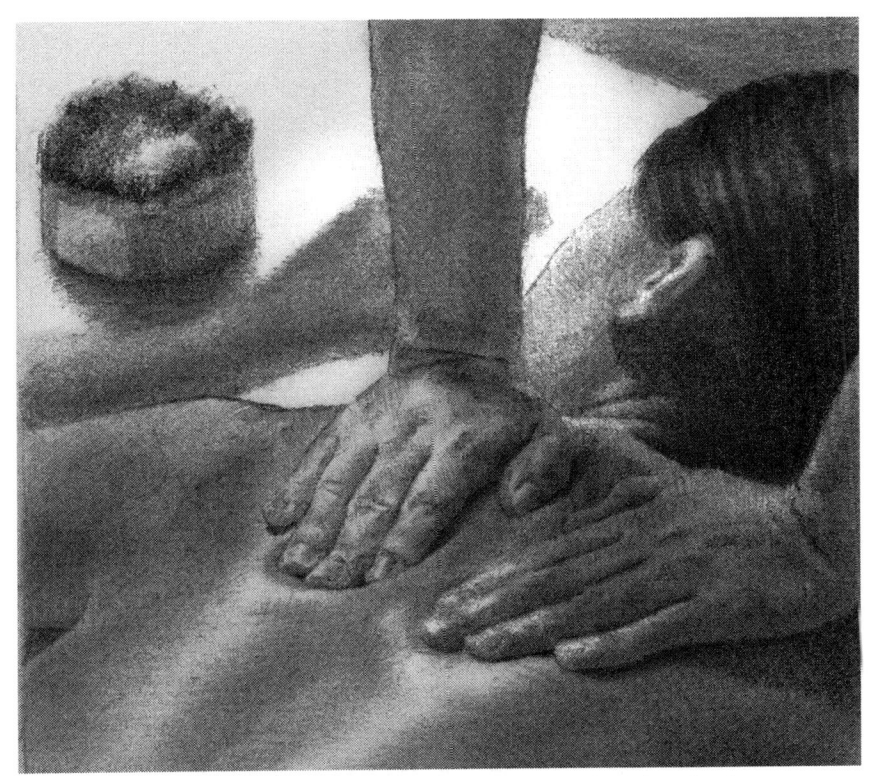

The nape should be massaged using your whole hand; place your hand with open palm on one side of the nape

- Use warm oil, and start your massage from the shoulders down, sliding your fingers along your partner's arms. Give special attention to the elbow, massaging it in a circular manner with the palm of your hand. The inner arm and legs are a very sensitive erogenous zones. Caress your Goddess's inner arm with the tips of your fingers and also with your tongue.

- Grasp your partner's wrist with your hand, encircling it with your fingers. Rotate your hand left and right. Lick her wrists, and then move to her palm and fingers. Take your time to lick each finger.

- Take each finger in your palm one at a time, close your hand, and gently rotate your fist left to right. Rub the heel of your palm against that of your partner's. This will strengthen your connection and facilitate the exchange of energy between the two of you.

Abdominal Massage

When performing an abdominal massage, you should try to use broad, unbroken motions, and treat the abdomen as a whole with your touches. Use massage oil, and ask your partner to lie on her back.

- Use both of your hands to cover as much of the abdominal area as possible. Keep your fingers together, and your hands should each follow the same rhythm.

- Imagine that your partner's abdomen is a butterfly, with its body extending from the pubis through the navel and to the solar plexus. Outline the butterfly's body with your hands, then trace its wings. Give them a different shape each time.

- For the lower abdomen, use a slow right-to-left motion beneath the navel. First, use both of your hands together to do this, and then let them move in opposite directions before meeting again.

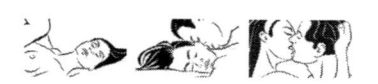

Exercise for Tantric Massage

Choose a night with your lover, and dedicate it to exploring the wonders of Tantric massage. Involve all of your senses in this process: Choose some sensual music, dim the lights, use some scented candles. Make sure that both you and your partner feel comfortable, and that you have plenty of uninterrupted time to explore the pleasures of massage. Use a massage oil of good quality, and warm it a little if necessary. Make sure your hands are clean and your nails cut. Have fun! Remember, the purpose of Tantric massage is to arouse both you and your partner, and to increase your sensuality. It is important to pay attention to your partner's needs and responses, and to adapt your massage techniques accordingly.

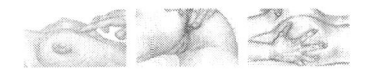

Motivational Moment

Tantric massage is a great way to explore your partner's body. It helps to build your connection, and it stimulates the sexual appetite. Tantric massage awakens the sacred kundalini energy and helps it circulate through your whole body, bringing balance and happiness into your life. Through Tantric massage, women often discover a new erogenous area(s) never stimulated before, and this opens a new level of sensuality and, often, a new intensity in her orgasm.

The Ancient Ritual of the Bath

The bath ceremony is known historically as a loving, nurturing ritual to promote physical, emotional, and spiritual healing. Women love to be recognized and given to freely, and a special bath will be a delicious experience for your lover. You can prepare a ritual bath for yourself; it can be a sumptuous gift from a partner, or it can be healing and replenishing experience for you and your partner to enjoy together. Bathing together is certainly a great form of mutual adoration—but generally, women feel more comfortable if they are clean before a sexual act.

Simply prepare a bath with warm water, sea salts, and a blend of carefully chosen organic oils; an excellent one on the market is called Erbaviva. You can learn specific ceremonial rituals and mantras for use when you are immersed in the water, which may make the bath more meaningful for you. Such a bath ceremony is overflowing with attuned focus and attention to each part of your body. It is the perfect complement to Tantric massage. Just make sure you have time and a secure setting for a safe haven before following the steps below for a luscious experience:

Prepare for the Bath

- Gather all of the oils, rose petals, candles, and any other ingredients you would like to enhance your bath, just as you did when preparing for Tantric massage.

- Draw the bath and prepare the warm water with sea salt, scented and skin-softening oils, a foaming agent or any other addition you or your partner would enjoy.

- Make sure time is plentiful and the setting secure.

- Remember to perform each part of the ritual with mindful awareness as this is a sacred time for you.

Begin the Bath Ceremony

- Remove your clothing in a slow manner, and begin to notice sensations as your nude body is exposed to air.

- Tenderly immerse yourself in the bath water.
- Make note of even the slightest physical and emotional sensations as you enter the water.

Mantra

A mantra is a repetition of certain syllables or words in a manner similar to repetitively saying a prayer. The goal of using a mantra is to open up your spiritual heart. If affirmations or some type of spiritual practice speak to you, this may be a way to create a bath ritual that has special meaning.

- If you wish, you can create and use your own affirmation, prayer, or mantra for the bath ceremony. Or you can obtain a Vedic, Hindu, or Buddhist book of mantras for ceremonial baths.
- Remember, it is vital that the invocation be for you because this bath ceremony is for you.

Breathing

Breathing deeply can enhance relaxation and eliminate any residual anxieties. The information below may aid in the discovery of the benefits of the complete breath. Initially, try to do at least two deep breaths, and increase the number as you feel comfortable.

- Be compassionate with yourself as you are developing skills.
- Exhale to allow the air to decrease in your abdominal area.
- Inhale, in a slow manner counting to ten.
- Hold your breath for a count of ten.
- Release your breath as you count to ten.

- Repeat.

Bath Massage

As the ritual progresses, the awareness of touch, release, or stimulation of each body part becomes apparent. If this beautiful present is given by a partner, the practice will be to receive the bath massage. If this is a self-organized practice, bath massage will be a delicious discovery of the various responses to touch in each part of the body. Here are some hints:

- Use some scented liquid soap, and pour a generous amount of onto your hands.

- Begin to touch and massage your (or your partner's) body, starting with the neck.

- Focus inward, and if you feel the slightest bit of anxiety, take a complete deep breath.

- Moving to your chest, caress you full breast and nipple.

- Notice the sensations of hands on your breasts with varying degrees of pressure.

- Move hands down over the abdomen, lower back, and buttocks, focusing on the release of stress and hints of arousal.

- Move back to the front of the body to the inner thighs and gently stroke the clitoral area.

- Gently slide hand over the vagina, parting the lips and tenderly stroking the inner lips leading into the vaginal canal.

- Allow yourself to feel the arousal, and let your body take the lead, possibly to orgasms.

- Follow down the legs and toes as well as the hands and feet.

The Ceremonial End

When your bathing is done, let yourself relax and soak. Treat yourself as mindfully at the end as in the beginning of the bath. The blood flow has been stimulated and the senses revitalized. When you are ready,

- Slowly exit the bath.
- Dry body gently with a thick towel.
- Put on a comfortable robe.
- Lie down and reflect on your experience.

Exercise about Setting the Atmosphere and Bath Ceremony

Surprise your lover tonight! Your home will be in complete darkness and the floor lit by many red candles, leading the way to your bath. Your partner will follow the candlelight to your bath, where more candles are lit all around. A vague scent of sweet perfume will float in the air like a delicate wisp of cirrus cloud in a bright-blue sky, present but barely perceptible. You will invite your lover to join you. Once the ceremonial bath is over, he will follow you to your bedroom, where incense and candles burn. You will lie down on your stomach, and whisper in his ear, "I would like to be erotically massaged and softly teased. I need you to take the time to listen to my body and how it responds. No big rush, just enjoy it."

Motivational Moment

Engaging in the Ceremonial Bath will definitely help with practicing more deeply several Tantric skills that can be put into practice in many aspects of the awakening of total physical, emotional, and spiritual awareness. Specific benefits include:

- Developing a deeply meditative state.
- Progressing in breathing skills.
- Awakening the senses.
- Freeing the mind and body of limitations and blockages.

The Erogenous Zones

Christine came to my office few days prior to our meeting. We had planned a session during which I would teach her to breathe deeply, faster and faster, while doing some Kegel exercises. She wanted to learn more about her body's different erogenous zones and which parts would initiate orgasm for her, so she wanted to be ready.

On the day of the meeting, Christine was waiting for me. The door was open, and she stood at the bottom of the stairs, wearing a negligee. Its black satin clung to her skin, her nipples clearly visible through the paper-thin material, which was cut so low that her areolas were visible over the top.

"I'm so glad you're here. I can't wait for you to massage me. I wanted so badly to touch myself all day, but I forced myself to wait," she told me as she reached out, looking to take my hands and lead me upstairs like a lover.

"I'm here now," I told her. "You are a beautiful woman, sexy and sensual. I can feel it, and I will help you achieve your deepest wishes with my massage."

We went upstairs, to a large master bedroom with walls painted a delicate lilac color. Incense sticks were burning in the corner. The centerpiece of the room was the king-size bed that provided not only acres of space, but also the ultimate in comfort.

Christine turned to face me, but I made the first move before she could even speak. I slipped the straps of her lingerie from her chocolate shoulders, feeling how smooth her skin was to my touch. The wispy material fell to the floor, and her nipples hardened instantly in the cool air of the bedroom. I reached out and stroked her erect body with the back of my hand, leaning in and lowering her to the bed in the process.

"You have a stunning body. I am honored to be able to touch you," I cooed into her ear. Her breathing was already beginning to increase, and her body shook as she exhaled.

"Just try to relax," I told her. Gently, I massaged her chest with my hands—, not just her breasts, but her entire upper body, I massaged her shoulders, feeling her need for release built up throughout her body.

"You body is a temple, and you are a Goddess. Lie back and relax," I encouraged her,

I began to gently massage Christine's delicate feet. It was obvious that she loved her feet, which were well cared for. But everything really started for Christine when I brought a toe to my mouth and licked under her feet. She could not really control herself any longer. Her hips begin to move up and down. For Christine, it was a beautiful revelation to have her feet licked.

The largest sensual organ is the skin. Erogenous zones are sexually sensitive areas of that great organ. Some parts of a woman's body are more sensitive to touch than others. Lips and labia, tongue, breasts, and nipples usually are the most responsive.

Yes, of course we all know about the millions of nerve endings in her breasts, vagina, and buttocks, but there are millions of others throughout her body. Touching these gently will awaken all of her, as you'll see.

Earlobe and Nape of the Neck

The earlobes and nape of the neck also can trigger sexual arousal. Take the time to nibble a bit on each ear lobe, and then move to the nape of her neck.

Kiss a woman's neck at the nape, and watch the frisson that you receive as a reaction! Kissing her clavicle also lets her know how special all of her is to you.

Hairline

Women spend hours on their hair, thus when you caress their hair, mentally this ties in with being cared for and the luxuriousness of her hair under your touch. She will feel tingles down her spine if you but outline her hairline delicately.

Small of the Back

You'd be totally surprised to hear women talk with one another about the exciting moment when a man touched the small of her back (lower back) when leading her through a crowd or directing her through an open door. Later, when she's nude, kiss her there, and you'll love the reaction.

Palm

The palm is seemingly such an innocuous place to touch, yet it is filled with nerve endings that sense the lightest of touches from your fingers or your lips as you kiss the insides of her hands. Kissing her palm is to arouse a flame that will not burn out for a long, long time!

Inner Thigh

This area usually rates as a perfect tease center for most women. Granted, it's difficult to kiss and lick her there and not venture upward to her vagina, but restraint here will bless you with even more excitement later on.

Hint for Men

To find your partner's erogenous zones, gently explore your partner's body with a light, subtle touch. Observe as she becomes aroused.

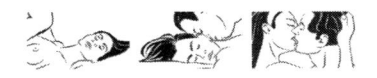

Exercise about the Erogenous Zones

When exploring an erogenous area, the secret is to keep an open mind. Let yourself be surprised by a touch or a kiss in a place that you never thought of as being erogenous, like your knee or elbow. Be playful, and turn it into a game by involving chance. Write on little pieces of paper the names of different areas of your body, and then fold them and put them in a container. With your partner, take turns extracting the slips of paper one by one, taking time to stimulate each other in that area before drawing another slip. No cheating or shortcuts: Try every area. You can use any means of stimulation that you like, from objects (a scarf or a feather) to the hands, mouth, and other body parts. Sometimes, you may find yourself laughing and at other times aroused. Just explore, and see what the game brings you.

Write a list of your erogenous zones as well as all of the unexplored parts of your body that you wish to investigate. I am sure you will find many ideas by reading this book! Tonight, talk about your list with your husband or partner, and then see if you decide to explore more. I am sure that there is some part of you that he never thought of touching that you would love for him to try. If you are single at this moment, this could be a nice way of starting a conversation with your next lover: "Tell me, darling, what is the most sensitive part of your body? Besides your penis—yes, I know that already!". Then he will ask you, and you will have a chance to explain your own magic spots.

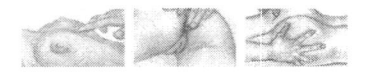

Motivational moment

Enticing and teasing the erogenous zones can improve the quality of orgasms. When erogenous parts of a woman's body are stimulated, her arousal builds. Her focus turns to the stimulation. She gets lost, in the end, in the experience of being kissed, licked, and touched.

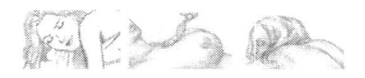

Note about Tantric Massage, Ceremonial Bath, and Erogenous Zones

In this chapter, you learned how to bring pure sensual pleasure into your life, and found out many how-to tips for performing a Tantric massage on your partner from head to toe. This chapter is addressed both to women who want to explore their erogenous areas and to men who want to offer their partners the gift of sensual bliss.

You also learned about the role of the Ceremonial Bath in learning to accept sensual pleasure and pay attention to your body's sensations.

This is useful, since the chapter went on to explain how to discover the erogenous zones of your body, as well as how to go from there to blossom and become a fully erogenous creature.

Fill out this log to keep a record of your results:

1. Which of these Tantric massage exercises did you do this week: Setting up the atmosphere? Bath ceremony? Exploring the erogenous zones? Use a feather or your mouth to stimulate erogenous areas of the head, breast, legs, arms, hands, anus, pelvic area?

2. What change do you want to see in yourself spiritually and sexually?

3. How do you feel about your own sexuality now you have done these exercises?

4. On a scale of 1 to 10, with 10 the maximum, how have these exercises improved the quality of your orgasm(s)?

	1	2	3	4
Week 1				
Week 2				
Week 3				
Week 4				
Week 5				
Week 6				
Week 7				
Week 8				

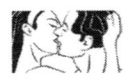

CHAPTER 4

Anatomy of the Yoni

Yoni, in Sanskrit, is the word for the genitals of a woman. I have noticed that most people believe that, for women, the clitoris is the seat of pleasure, and that orgasms begin and eventually end there. Actually, the entire female body is the seat of pleasure, and of course, the entire female body is involved in both orgasm and the end of the orgasm, when a sense of satisfaction takes over.

The reason why we need to be utterly familiar with the vulva and breasts (and the penis!—see Chapter 11) is that we all search for better orgasms. Yes, orgasms feel good. At times they shake our entire world, but at other times they just lie there or only gently shake us, much as a mother rocks a sleeping infant. What makes the difference, we wonder, and why should one orgasm be just "okay" and another rate as a "10"? Some question if there is a "10" at all. Does a "10" orgasm only happen to "other women," and what do those other women, or their lovers, do differently?

I have met women who could achieve a hundred orgasms during sexual intercourse and others who could achieve none. This book is meant as an opportunity for you to give yourself every chance to have better orgasms. This is why it addresses both women and their partners, since the openness, knowledge, and understanding of both are crucial to achieving single and multiple orgasms.

Many areas of the female body can lead to orgasm. When a lover finds these spots, the result is incredible climaxes that seem to roll from one into the other. This happens when a lover—and ladies, this includes yourselves—knows enough about a particular woman to bring her to such pleasures.

The Mons Pubis

When you first view a female without clothing, you will see that she has a fatty mound above her pubic bone. This is normal, regardless of the rest of her body's makeup. The mound is there to protect her pubic bone during sex. The mound will have pubic hair on it unless she's shaved it; this is common today, although some males and females prefer that the hair remains.

A soft touch is best for the mound. When hair remains, slight pulling turns some women on; if shaved, the mound can be kissed and licked gently. The mons pubis is a highly erogenous zone for some women, but unfortunately, many men are not aware of this fact and miss out on a great opportunity for excitement.

The Clitoris: The Crown Jewel

In looking at the female body, most are intrigued by the clitoris, that little jewel found between a woman's legs in what is known as the vulva. The vulva encompasses all of the sexual organs, which are made of tissues that are tremendously rich in both blood vessels and nerve endings.

The clitoris is called the "Crown Jewel" in the Tantric world. If you part the lips of the vulva, you will see that the clitoris is positioned at the very top of the female genitals. This is why we are describing the clitoris next, as it is directly below the mound. (*see drawing: If you part the lips of the vulva, you will see that the clitoris is positioned at the very top of the female genitals)*

The size of a woman's clitoris has no bearing on how much pleasure she can receive, since it is loaded with more than eight thousand nerve endings! The roots of these are located in the G-spot, or Skene's glands. All women have the exact same number of nerve endings, regardless of the size of their clitoris; although men may worry whether "size matters," women do not need to have such uncertainty.

The clitoris is very similar to a man's penis as far as sexual sensitivity is concerned. Keep in mind, however, that the clitoris, unlike the penis, does not have an opening to allow urine or ejaculate to pass through. A woman's urethra is found in the vulva but is not accessible via the clitoris at all. Unlike the male's penis, the female's clitoris is present only to allow women to attain sexual pleasure: That's how special it is. Note too that the clitoris is not just that little nub, called the glans clitoris, but that much of the clitoris's body is actually buried within the vaginal opening. What is visible is but the very tiny tip of the clitoris.

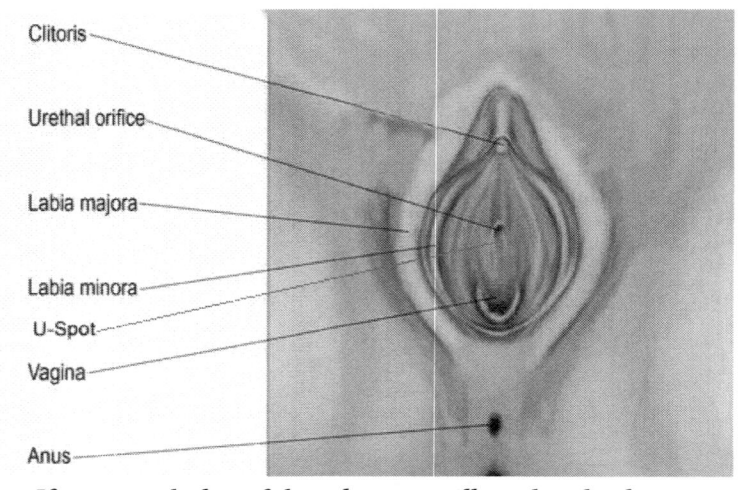

If you part the lips of the vulva, you will see that the clitoris is positioned at the very top of the female genitals

Some women are more sensitive than others around their clitoral area. Women who have a prominent clitoris receive a lot of clitoral pleasure when made love to in what most people call the "missionary position"—the man on top of the woman between her parted legs–but this is not so with every woman. In order for a woman to experience a clitoral orgasm, her clitoris usually needs varying amounts of direct stimulation. Each woman is different: Some like to be touched gently and lightly, others with a harder touch and more pressure. Because something works with one woman does not mean that it will work with all of them. So many times women say to me, "He doesn't listen to me and stimulates me all over the place," or "His touch is too hard," or "I need a softer motion." A man should become aware of the effect he has on his partner by becoming one with her. Then he will become a great lover.

How a woman likes to have her clitoris touched is completely independent of how orgasmic she is or may become. Regardless of what kind of touch a woman desires, it's up to her partner to match what she says is best. Whether using the penis, the hand, or the mouth and lips, it behooves the man to explore her tenderly to find out what she likes and dislikes, keeping in mind that every woman is different.

The Shaft

The shaft of the clitoris, measuring about 1½ inches in length, has spongy tissue like the penis and may erect under stimulation. The shaft is attached to the pubic bone; on each side are two legs, the crura (or crus, if referring to only one), measuring about 3 inches, which are attached to the base of the pubis.

The entire clitoris looks like an upside-down letter 'Y' that has been bent forward at the top. It is covered by a foreskin (or prepuce or hood). When a woman is sexually aroused, the clitoris swells slightly, the foreskin pulls back, and the glans or "button," which is the most sensitive part of the clitoris, becomes hard. This is similar to what happens when a penis becomes erect when stimulated. Internally, the clitoral shaft has a little bend in it, called the "clitoral knee." If you imagine it as a crooked finger, only the top joint emerges from the foreskin.

Unlike the shaft of the penis, which hangs freely, the clitoris is fixed in place beneath the skin, and so a woman has little freedom of motion for stimulation. The penis's ability to move enables a man to thrust in and out of his partner; if the penis were fixed like the clitoris, a man would need to rub his body up and down along his partner's body to stimulate himself in the same way that a woman rubs up and down against his pubic bone.

It may sound as though women are at a disadvantage because of the clitoris's inability to move; however, this is not true. Since the clit is fixed in place, any downward pull on the skin covering the shaft and forks of the clitoris is felt directly in the glans. This means that a penis going in and out of the vagina, indirectly stimulates the glans clitoris by pulling and releasing the clitoral root and shaft. This indirect stimulation can often cause a woman to have an orgasm, even though it may take longer than having an orgasm by direct stimulation of the clit. Since the clitoris is covered by skin and fat, many men and women think that they have not stimulated the clitoris when in fact they have done so.

A vaginal orgasm is actually an orgasm produced by the clitoral crura. Although these types of orgasms occur, they are less common than those produced by direct stimulation of the clitoris. This is because male ejaculation usually happens before the crura have been sufficiently excited. However; a female ejaculation which is issue from the stimulation of the Skene's gland is not a vaginal orgasm.

The Labia Majora and Minora

Some women have prominent labia, or lips, surrounding the vagina, and some have very withdrawn or tiny labia; keep in mind that all are normal, regardless of the predominance of one type or the other.

The lips themselves can be tenderly rubbed and gently pulled apart to locate the vagina, as well as the clitoris. (*see drawing: The lips themselves can be tenderly rubbed*) Any—and the emphasis is on *any*—of these parts can be gently licked to bring untold pleasure to the female. Partners, take your time: At the beginning, lick slowly. You will notice the whole vulva getting darker and swelling when your partner approaches a certain level of excitement leading up to her orgasm.

The Urethral Opening

The urethra, located just above the vagina, can provide a place for bacteria to grow and become infected. It is important for a woman to urinate after intercourse to prevent infection.

The Vagina

The vagina, in Sanskrit, is called the "Sacred Temple" or "Divine Passage." This is the orifice that will be used for entry, whether by a tampon, penis, tongue, or hand. The vagina is also where a baby comes from when a woman gives birth. The vagina is tremendously elastic, as it needs to be able to accept a penis or the fingers of a hand and, ultimately, a baby's head.

The vagina is also the marvelous passageway between the vulva and the cervix (*see drawing: The advantages of stronger PC muscles are several and all highly desirable: absolutely and affirmatively better orgasms*) or the neck of the uterus, found very deep inside. The vagina itself can be pleasured by penis, tongue, or fingers, and if additional wetness is needed to pleasure other sections of a woman's vulva, this is where it can be obtained. A larger penis will occasionally push upon the cervix, which some women find erogenous and some others do not enjoy.

The G-Spot

Inside the vagina, located in its frontal wall (on the roof or upper side when a woman is lying on her back), is the famous "G-spot."

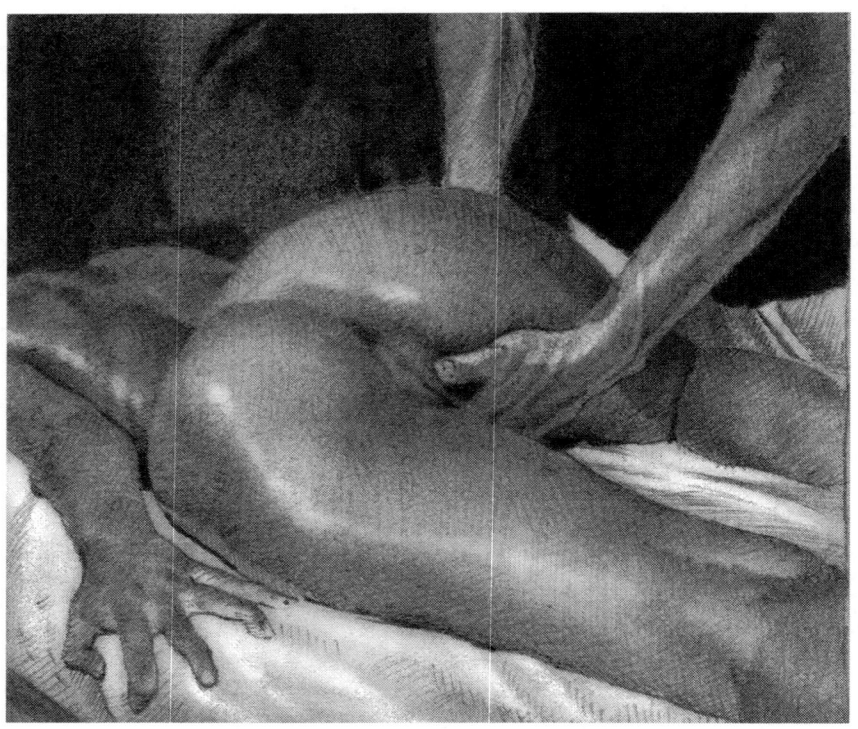

The lips themselves can be tenderly rubbed

The Gräfenberg spot, named after German gynecologist Ernst Gräfenberg, causes additional sexual pleasure, and its stimulation can result in female ejaculation ("Amrita" in Sanskrit). The G-spot is located approximately 1½ inches from the opening of the vagina, has a ridged structure much like the roof of the mouth, or buccal cavity, and under stimulation increases in size. G-spot pleasure is probably the greatest pleasure a woman will encounter, and I would encourage any woman to explore this. I have met women who have never experienced orgasm from stimulation of the clitoral area but who have tremendous ejaculations. Later on, they found they were able to experience pleasure from the clitoral area. Our senses are in continuous evolution, and it is important to leave open all of the doors, to be able to experience new, unexpected pleasures.

The Pubococcygeus Muscles

Whether you are eighteen years old or seventy, as a woman you are going to need your pubococcygeus muscles. All around the vagina a woman has a tremendous amount of muscular tissue, and it is these muscles that tighten and loosen during the act of having sex and during orgasm. No wonder these PC muscles are also known as the love muscles.

The pubococcygeus muscles may be strengthened by tightening them with Kegel exercises (see Chapter 7). In addition to performing traditional Kegels, some different ways to improve the strength of the PC muscles include toys or exerciser aids such as jade or Ben Wa balls, barbells, or the Kegelmaster. (*see pictures: Ben Wa balls, barbells, the Kegelmaster*) The advantage of using a device inside the vagina is that the muscles automatically know what to do, and exercising this way will make the muscles stronger than if you exercise the PC muscles consciously without squeezing anything. The metal or jade balls are great because of their weight, and they can be used discreetly during the day to strengthen. (*see picture: metal balls*) With practice, stronger PC muscles may bring you to a vaginal orgasm. Wouldn't it be nice to have a very pleasant orgasm while you are working at your desk and smiling at your boss—something that 90 percent of women wish they could have?

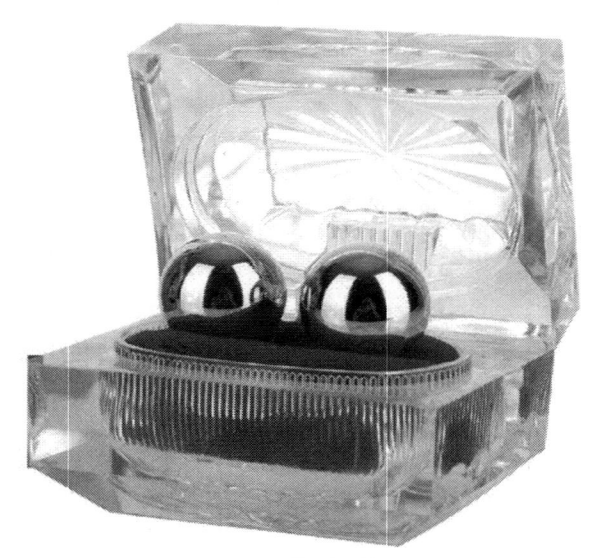

Ben Wa balls

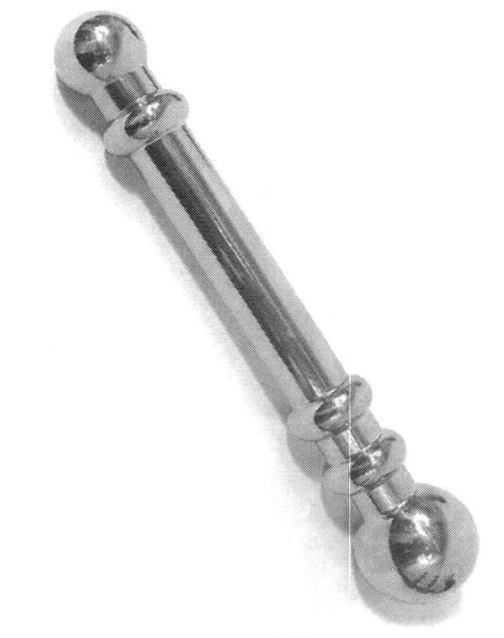

Barbells

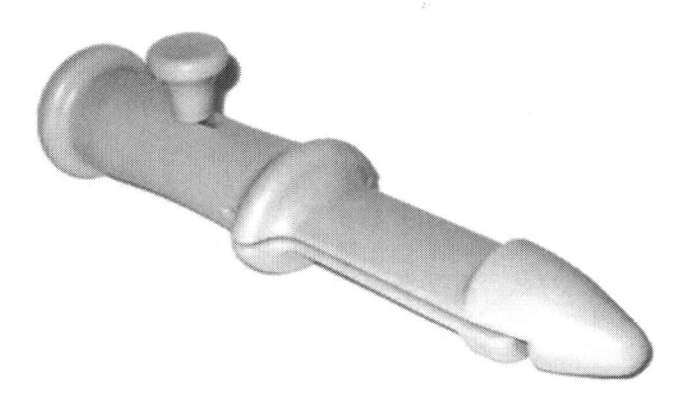

The Kegelmaster

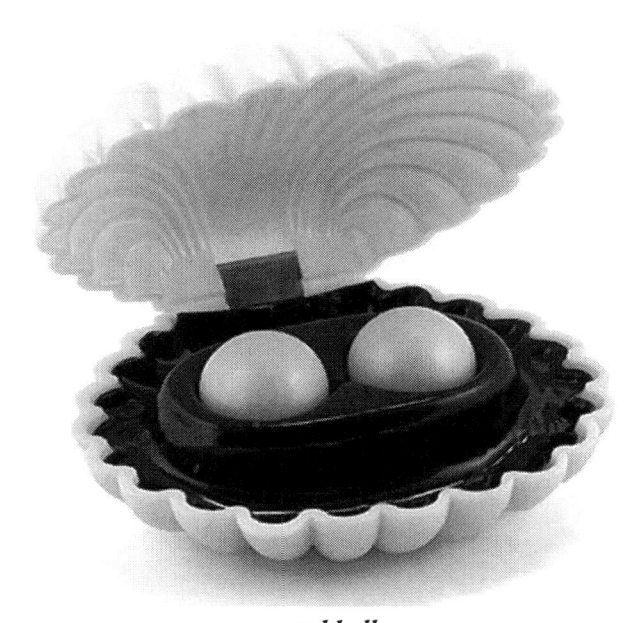

metal balls

The advantages of stronger PC muscles are several and all highly desirable: absolutely and affirmatively better orgasms, proper positioning of the fetus during delivery, and control of urinary continence, especially when estrogen levels fall with the approach of menopause. (*see drawing: The advantages of stronger PC muscles are several and all highly desirable: absolutely and affirmatively better orgasms*)

The A-Spot

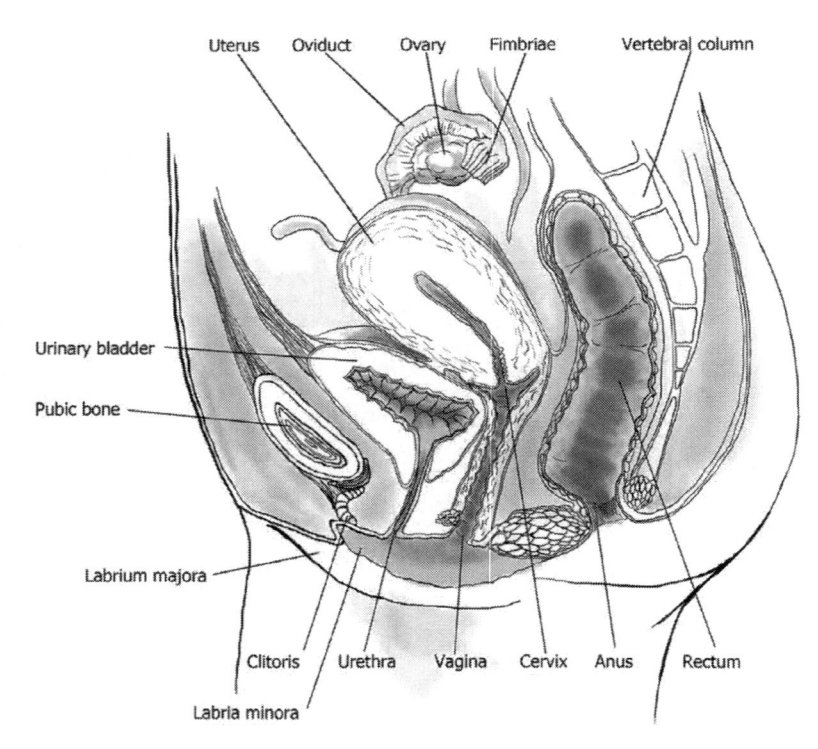

The advantages of stronger PC muscles are several and all highly desirable: absolutely and affirmatively better orgasms

The anterior fornix erogenous zone, discovered by the Malaysian Dr. Chua Chee Ann, is located deeper inside the vagina toward the uterus (*see drawing: The advantages of stronger PC muscles are several and all highly desirable: absolutely and affirmatively better orgasms;* and drawing: *Scientists increasingly call the Skene's glands the "female prostate" because they make secretions that are almost identical to the seminal fluid produced by the male prostate in Chapter 7*) and is known as the "A-spot." The A-spot is sometimes referred to as a secondary G-spot because it too can produce an orgasm if stimulated repeatedly, and it definitely creates ample vaginal lubrication or wetness in the female. The penis rarely reaches this spot because it is so deep within the vagina; however, the A-spot can be stimulated using the fingers or curved toys made specifically to reach it. As you can see from the diagram, it too is located on the upper portion of the vagina when a woman is lying on her back. For some women, the A-spot can be extremely pleasurable, especially if stimulated at the same time as the G-spot. Some women may have female ejaculation by massage of the A-spot alone. A-spot massage must be very gentle, unlike G-spot massage, which can be quite vigorous.

The U-Spot

This is the latest erogenous zone that has been discovered, and there have been many reports that gently rubbing this area, whether manually, penis or tongue, can create an orgasm. This erogenous zone is logically called the "U-spot" and is found directly above and to the sides of the urethra's opening. (*see drawing: The "U-spot" is found directly above and to the sides of the urethra's opening*)

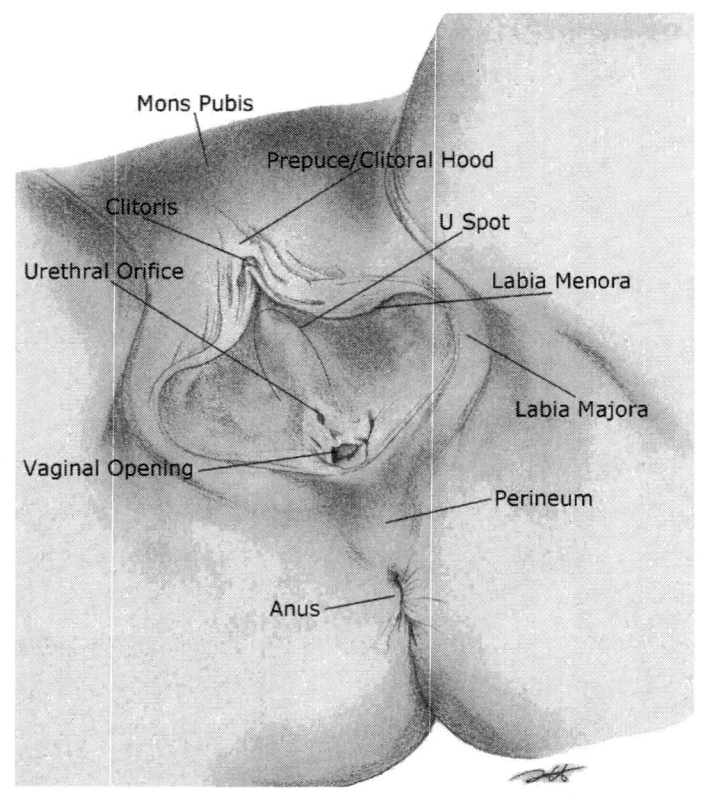

The "U-spot" is found directly above and to the sides of the urethra's opening

It needs to be stimulated gently, perhaps using the moisture of the vagina. Also ask your partner to rub with his tongue delicately in order to create pleasure. The U-spot is a jewel of secret pleasure, and you will love to receive some attention in that zone.

The Perinea

Finally, moving toward the anus, we encounter the perinea (*see drawing: The "U-spot" is found directly above and to the sides of the urethra's opening*), which is the area just in front of the anus. It is a highly sensitive area that has many nerve endings. This erogenous zone can be used to excite a woman with gentle touches, kisses, and licks of the tongue. I call the perinea my life buoy; if your partner does not respond to your other foreplay, pushing the perinea gently will do wonderful work for a man.

The Breasts

When a female is excited sexually, her body sends messages to her brain telling it to increase blood flow to her sexual organs. As a result, a woman's entire vulva becomes very moist and fully engorged with blood. Similarly, the breasts begin to swell, which makes the nipples harden.

The more this happens, the more sensitive a woman becomes to touch, and so the brain is told to send more blood into these areas. In essence, this is why women are slower to fully excite: This loop of pleasurable messaging from the body to the brain and from the brain to blood flow needs to be sent forth a number of times for complete sexual excitement.

Female breasts are often the means to sexual excitation. Medically, the breasts are referred to as mammary glands, but sexually there are many different names associated with female breasts. Of course, you know that female breasts are responsible for milk production after a female gives birth. Sexually, however, the breast has many nerve endings, especially around the nipple and the darker portion called the areola. When excited sexually, a woman's nipples harden, and the skin around them puckers.

Breasts come in a variety of sizes, of course, but size does not affect the sensual feelings of the breast. Every woman derives different pleasures from having her breasts touched or sucked, and the pleasure triggers are different from woman to woman.

Caressing the female breast can mean just that—gentle soft touches—while some women prefer a harder touch such as kneading or pinching of the breast area and the nipple. Exploration of a woman's breasts is one of the joys of sex for both man and woman.

Correspondence with the Penis/Lingam

The penis, or *lingam* in Sanskrit, is the male organ. In Tantra, it is useful to remember that its parts correspond to women's anatomy as follows:

- Clitoris = Head of penis
- Hood = Foreskin
- Labia Majora = Scrotum
- Labia Minora = Shaft
- Ovaries = Testicles
- Perinea = Perinea
- Anus = Anus.

The lingam is discussed in full detail in Chapter 11.

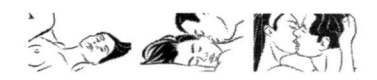

Anatomy Exercise for Women and Men

This chapter is not meant merely to be a course in anatomy. The point is to use your knowledge. People often take small, halting steps on the path to full sexual awareness. Letting go in a Tantric way requires practice. Here are a few exercises you can try:

- Place your naked self in front of a mirror, and learn about your body. Study the entire genital area. It is important to slowly discover your body, focusing and meditating on each part of the anatomy described above. Become aware of their form and the pleasure it can give you. The more you become aware of your sexual anatomy, the more you will enjoy.

- Look at the vaginal lips. Part them, and see the wonderful pink tissues that you have.

- Next, locate your clitoris, your urethra, your vagina, the perinea, and your anus. Don't just look; ever so gently touch them all, explore, and be amazed.

- Caress your breast and nipples and watch their color changing and how hard and erect they become.

- Caress your clitoris and watch the physical changes that occur.

- You also may do the same for your partner and let your partner do the same for you. You may take his penis, caress it and stroke it but don't make him ejaculate. He will do the same for your breast, vagina, labias and clitoris, Becoming aware of each other's sexual anatomy is a good way to get to know each other and increase the sexually trust between you. This practice can be done each time prior to sex. It may feel awkward at first, but you will start to feel more and more comfortable with each other and his/her body very rapidly. Trusting each other is the first step for an amazing orgasm.

Motivational Moment

The nicest and best way to learn more about what your body can bring you, and how to have better orgasms with each sexual adventure, is to know where everything is located (including your U-spot, G-spot, and A-spot), how deeply your glans clitoris goes, and (even better) how to stimulate them! Exploration of all your magic spots is the best way to start your sexual journey. Do not expect your partner to always be able to pleasure you if you yourself do not know everything about your anatomy. You should be able to communicate with and guide him so that you will have wonderful sexual pleasure together.

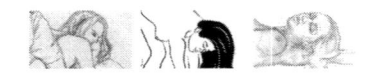

Note About Sexual Anatomy

This chapter has pointed out all of the erogenous zones that you will encounter throughout this book. You will undoubtedly return to this chapter again and again for clarification, as these zones will be used as your pleasure spots for better and better orgasms.

Fill in this log to record the results of your exercises:

1. Which of your magic spots did you explore this week: Mons Pubis, Clitoris, A-Spot, U-Spot, G-spot, Vagina, Perinea, Breasts? Did you do your Kegels or try exercise aids for strengthening your PC muscles?

2. What change do you want to see in yourself spiritually and sexually?

3. How do you feel about your own sexuality, now that you have done these exercises?

4. On a scale of 1 to 10, with 10 the maximum, how have these exercises improved the quality of your orgasm(s)?

	1	2	3	4
Week 1				
Week 2				
Week 3				
Week 4				
Week 5				
Week 6				
Week 7				
Week 8				

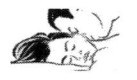

CHAPTER 5

Romancing the Yoni

When a woman is passionate about learning Tantra massage, the connection is passionate with a sense of urgency. One such e-mail came into my inbox. It was from a woman called Mizuuki. With the Japanese name, I was immediately intrigued and opened her e-mail to read it:

"I know it's short notice," Mizuuki wrote, *"but I picked up your business card at Starbucks. I am looking for massage tonight. I was originally going for Shiatsu massage in my area, but since I checked your website, I think I have to give Tantric massage a try. If you can get back to me with your availability, it would be wonderful."*

For a moment I paused. A Shiatsu massage was far different from a Tantric massage. Tantric massage is passionate and warm, whereas Shiatsu massages the deep tissues. I sent Mizuuki a short message: *"I trust you are aware there is a difference in these two types of massages. Please tell me what you are interested in about the massage, and send a phone number so we can discuss this further."*

I sat and waited for her response, wondering for a moment if the nature of Tantric massage would turn her off rather than entice her to come forward looking for more.

"I need a sensual, erotic massage," came her immediate reply." I expect a general feeling of being appreciated, with lots of foreplay. In our culture, men do not understand that women love to be orally stimulated from head to toes. We Japanese women are extremely erotic, but men are far more direct in matters of sexuality and do not appreciate the pleasure to be teased."

As I began driving down the road, I checked my GPS to avoid the traffic going into Pasadena. When I came to Mizuuki's apartment, the thought crossed my mind that she must have felt so very brazen meeting me on such short notice. She'd worn her favorite kimono for me, as she'd said she would over the phone. She said that the silk material felt like soft kisses with every minute movement as it brushed against her shaven parts and her nipples.

The moment Mizuuki answered the door, her very eyes spoke to me. I saw her as she really was: a young, very sophisticated Japanese woman who, in a moment, was about to offer herself to my ministrations. As Mizuuki led me to her bedroom, I never once commented on the beautiful apartment. I knew from our earlier conversation what awaited me— her pure yet incredible sexual need—thus I felt no need for idle chitchat.

After I set up my potions and oils next to her bed, Mizuuki turned toward me. Brazenly, she came to me and put her arms around me. Once the embrace was over, she did another very brazen thing: She asked me to undress her. Over the phone, she'd told me that her kimono had been a gift from her father long ago for her "coming of age day," when she was a teenager, and that she only wore it for special occasions. I had been unsure, up until that moment, just what a special occasion this was.

The heavy pale-green silk robe was painstakingly hand decorated with sprays of dark cherry-tree blossoms. When I pulled on the sash clip, releasing the obi scarf from its neat folds and tucks, I heard her utter a small gasp, and because I knew what my undressing her meant in her culture, I found it utterly charming.

Mizuuki turned to me completely naked, and my eyes grew wide for a moment. I'd never seen such a beautiful Japanese woman before, and I knew that she could see the appreciation in my eyes. Indeed, my eyes were already caressing her sensuous and lithe physique.

I reached for her and stroked her back with long, coursing touches that promised such bliss to her that I could tell her sensual interest burgeoned with each stroke. As she sank to the mattress, her last words were, "Give me your ultimate best oral massage. . . ."

Introduction to Analingus

Oral sex involving the anal area, or analingus, has often been touted as absolutely incredible.

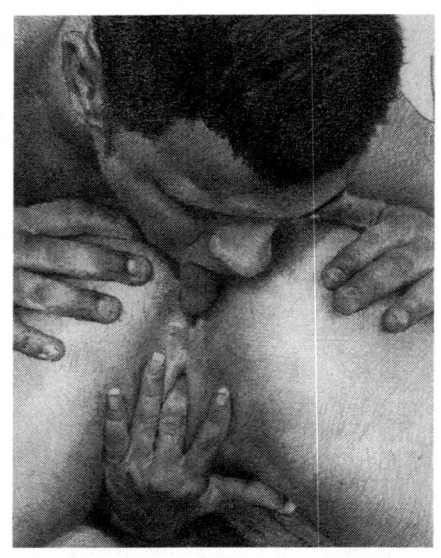

Only a bit of mental acceptance and relaxation is needed to experience its amazing pleasure

The reason why it is considered so exciting and pleasurable is that there are so many fascinating, ultrasensitive nerve endings around the anal opening and its surrounds, including the perinea. In my latest quiz 85% of women absolutely love to have their ass licked. It is taboo, but women find it delicious.

Many women will not consider having their mate perform analingus on them because of the age-old puritanical taboo surrounding the practice. A few years back, every state in the United States had a law against oral sex, and yet today it is widely accepted and is considered a normal sexual practice. So it is with analingus: Only a bit of mental acceptance and relaxation is needed to experience its amazing pleasures. (*see drawing: Only a bit of mental acceptance and relaxation is needed to experience its amazing pleasures*)

On the other hand, analingus may be extra exciting in part because of the mysterious taboo around it. We humans seem to have a predilection for the taboo. When we partake in taboo sex practices that intrigue us, they test our boundaries; we press beyond our comfort zones, opening up a new set of pleasures.

Some women are introduced to analingus when their mates perform cunnilingus or ordinary oral sex on them; when a woman is sufficiently turned on, her partner may begin to slip down from the vulva and into the anal area with his mouth and tongue. This is a gentle way of introducing analingus into your love life, as opposed to discussing it and plunging in directly, which tends to raise the embarrassment factor. This is not to say that analingus should not be discussed; just the opposite is actually true. Making it less of a clinical experiment, however, will go far in enabling you to accept it as normal.

The Physical Act

Physically, the act of analingus is exciting as it involves manipulation of the pelvic floor (PC) muscles, which occurs naturally when the anal area is sexually excited. Interestingly, these same muscles eventually will contract rather violently when you reach orgasm.

The Emotional Act

There is a tremendous amount of "emotional meaning" behind analingus for both the person performing it and the person receiving it. First, it takes a huge amount of trust on your part as the receiver. How wonderful it is to be so open to another person and to trust them with such a personal and highly protected physical zone.

A giver of analingus conveys a message of extreme closeness to the receiver; no area is barred, and nothing about the partner is a turnoff! Your partner may refuse to receive analingus today, but she may be very open to the idea tomorrow. Regardless of the reaction you receive, don't be discouraged and continue to be gently adventurous; she will always be thankful for it.

Protective Measures

If you partner wants to feel more protected, analingus can be performed through dental dams to avoid bacteria, or a sheer glyde dams which is silky thin sheet of scented latex or you can even use ordinary plastic food wrap. You will feel more of the tongue and mouth if lubricant is utilized to heighten pleasure. This method will also prevent bacteria infection to the vagina.

Suggested Positions

Having the receiver positioned on knees and elbows is highly recommended; also, lying on the back with knees against the chest opens up the anal area marvelously if a pillow is placed under the recipient's hips.

Important Tips

Above all else, just as in all sexual acts, it is best to go slow and be deliberate. The anus is a highly sensitive area that should not just be "attacked."

Utilizing massage techniques, slow kisses, and soft licks to the general area, work gradually toward the anus and make sure the receiver is as relaxed as possible. The anticipation alone is highly erotic! I have always taken an extraordinary amount of time with these suggested preliminaries, which arouses the female to splendid proportions.

There are times when your partner should make the tongue soft and flat, exerting the least amount of pressure, and then change to harder pressure, alternating between the two. By pointing the tongue your partner can rim the outside of the hole with quite a bit of pressure, and finally, insert the tongue as far into the hole as possible. At the risk of being repetitive, GO SLOWLY!

Perinea

While we are in the general area, remember that the perinea, located between the entrance to the vagina and the anal area, is a great help if, after extended foreplay, your partner is still not aroused. Some soft stimulation either with your finger or your tongue will make intercourse much more pleasant for the receiver. The stimulation of the perinea saved me more than once of a very dry vagina. This area has a nerve center that runs all the way through the genital region and is largely responsible for the conduction of intense pleasure signals. When a partner touches, kisses, and licks this area, you will find that it greatly aids the engorgement of the whole genital area.

Analingus Exercise

As strange as it may feel to do this, you will find that you will learn a lot about how strongly analingus will affect you if you use lubrication or your wet finger to touch yourself in the anal area. Squat in front of a mirror and observe how every movement you make with the very tip of your finger makes you feel. It is such a sensitive area that every movement you make will feel wonderful. After this exercise, it will be easy to imagine what it will feel like when your lover does this to you.

Motivational Moment

Experimenting on yourself will awaken you to a new, exciting erogenous zone. You may then share this tremendously intimate experience with your lover. These new discoveries will forge a sense of complicity and a bond between you and your partner, since you now know that you can give each other these secret pleasures.

The Magic of Cunnilingus

The result of the personal quiz I sent to my clients at http://mysecretquiz.com/index.php

>   I receive oral stimulation 10 times out of 10 during foreplay: 33%

>   I receive oral stimulation 5 times out of 10 during foreplay: 29%

>   I never receive oral stimulation during foreplay: 7%

I have spoken to a great number of women, all of whom tell me that cunnilingus is one of the greatest pleasures that a lover can give to a woman. I have sent out hundreds of questionnaires, and most women report that they have far more orgasms as a result of clitoral stimulation than from vaginal penetration.

It is very unfortunate that some men shy away from cunnilingus, even if their women desire it. This may come from archaic misconceptions that cunnilingus is dirty or unclean—which certainly is not true, especially if you bathe prior to indulging. If you are a healthy female, a partner will describe the taste and smell of your vaginal juices as anywhere from incredibly delicious to tantalizingly sweet. I would tell men to get over their objections and to use buccal protection, for sale in all pharmacies, during cunnilingus if they like.

Unfortunately, some men agree to cunnilingus only as a means of being granted open passage to intercourse. They do not engage in it because they love it but, rather, for ulterior motives. Over and over again, I've been told by women that their principal frustration is that men perform the act for only a few minutes, and then it's all over. The most asked questions from these women is *"what should I do, how can I prevent to be disappointed by my next lover?"* I have only one advice for them. Before anything happens between you and your new lover, let him know that you wish to be orally pleasured and have your orgasm before he takes his own pleasure by penetrating you. Otherwise, he will never see you again. They all smile and said *"It is simple, I will say no next time"*.

The Lucky One

When a woman finds a man who is good at performing oral sex, she has found a treasure she will not let go of very easily. This is an exceedingly rare find, and she knows it all too well. In fact, she will not even share this information with her girlfriends, for fear her guy will become the most popular man in town. Let's face it: Most guys know how to penetrate a woman, and in general they do it satisfactorily; but the guy who can perform fantastic oral sex on a woman is a man she will hold close.

Oral sex is an art that is exceedingly similar to kissing a woman, and your partner will know from the very first touch if you are good at it or not. If you are good at it, your forehead will always be marked by that sign whenever she sees you.

I will never forget going one day to meet a woman who, on her bedside table, had the infamous book *She Comes First*. I picked up the book and looked at it, and that's when she told me, "*I ask each of my lovers to read that book prior to sleeping with me. The dear man who reads this particular book had best be good at cunnilingus as well as enjoy it.*"

She meant what she said, and no wonder. Oral sex is one of the greatest arts, which all women seek. It is an art because it is precise and very delicate. Women will love you for this talent if you have it, since most women can only achieve orgasm through clitoral stimulation. I have had some of the most beautiful women in Hollywood beg me for more due to my oral talent. If I can do this, so can you.

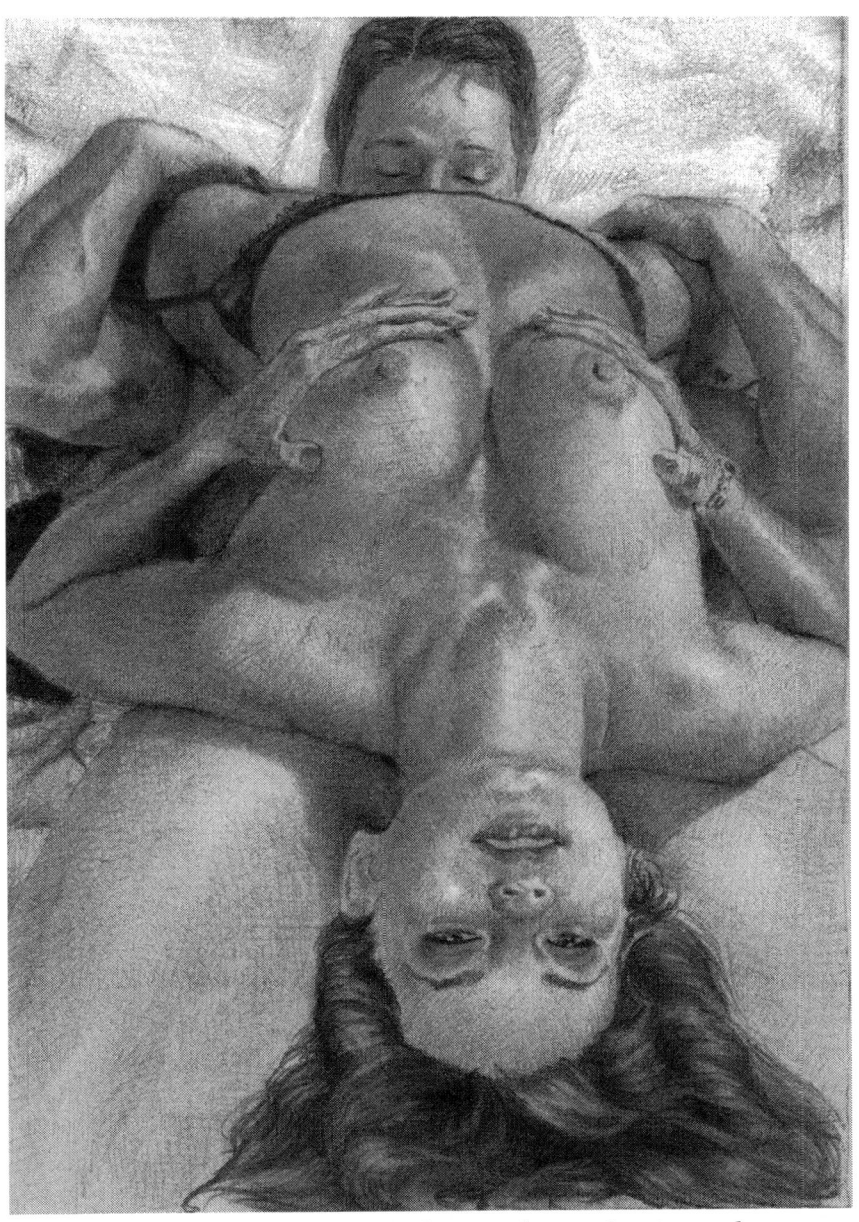

*When a woman finds a man who is good at performing oral sex,
she has found a treasure she will not let go of very easily*

Compliment Her

You will find that there is nothing that makes a woman more unique than her vulva. You will see that vulvas come in all different sizes, colors, and shapes. Some are tucked inside like a little girl's cunny, and some have thick, luscious lips that open out to greet you. Some are nestled in huge furry bushes, while others are barely covered with transparent fuzz. Be sure to appreciate the unique qualities of your woman's vulva, and tell her why she is special to you.

In general, women are a great deal more verbal than men, and this is especially so during lovemaking. Women also respond more to verbal love. This means that the more you talk to her, the easier it will be to arouse her. Throughout the time you are petting and stroking her stunning vulva, talk to her about it. Tell her how beautiful her jewel is, and admire it. Women love their vulvas so much that they often name them and often speak to them. This is part of the secret women's world.

Technique

Whenever you touch a woman's vulva, be sure that your finger is either wet or coated with a lubricant or gel made for this purpose. Of course, you can always lick your finger or use the juices from inside of her.

A clitoris, especially, needs to be wetted to touch it, as it does not have its own juices and is thus extremely sensitive. If your finger is dry, it will stick to the clitoris, and this will hurt. You are not yet ready to touch her clitoris, however; there are miles to go prior to this happening, and you have to work up to it.

You see, before she's completely aroused, a woman's clitoris is much too delicate to be handled. Approach her vulva slowly and imagine it as the most delicate flower in the world. And keep in mind that it will take some time before you can go inside.

At first, use your tongue to slowly lick the groin area, the two creases on either side of the pubic area where her legs join her torso. Lick the creases where her legs join her vulva, and then move on to another spot. Then go down and lick her perinea, this is the most sensitive part. The stimulation of the perinea will arouse her in no time. Then, if you are brave and want to really please your Goddess, lick her ass. She will know that you know well her most d secret desire and taboo. Above all, you must make her desire and anticipate.

She will love it if you nuzzle her bush with your entire face, and then brush your lips over her vulva ever so lightly without pressing down upon it to excite her. You want to use every means possible to tease her.

If she says that you are teasing her, more power to you, for you are doing it correctly. Women love a man who is a teaser, and you are going to make her beg for cunnilingus. Remember: Once you make her beg for it, she is yours.

At this point, she will try to bring her clitoris as close as possible to your tongue, but you will not allow that. You are much stronger than she is; you are her master, and you are there to win her over. Later on, she will let you know how much she appreciated this.

So, now it appears that you have her bucking up from her position, and she is straining to somehow make you get closer to her pleasure area; this is when you put your lips directly onto her vulva.

With your lips, you will barely brush and softly touch so very delicately the entire vulva, moving your lips up and down and back up again, taking all the time in the world. Do this for a few minutes, and then kiss her ever so gently. Then kiss her a bit harder. Using your tongue now, gently separate her lips, and as she opens to you, run your tongue gently up and down those layers of labial flesh. Everything must be done very slowly, as if you are savoring the moment, and of course, your touch must be very gentle.

Using only your tongue, gently pull the lips apart and look at the inner lips, licking these slowly and savoring them. You may now spread the very top of her vulva to look at her clitoris. You can use your lips and tongue to come tantalizingly close to the clitoris, but do not touch it yet.

As you view it, you'll realize that a woman's clitoris comes in varying sizes, just as males have different-sized penises. The size of her clitoris is meaningless as far as her capacity for orgasms. A very small clitoris only means that more of it is hidden under her hood. I have seen women whose very tiny clitorises brought them orgasms that lasted all night long, nonstop!

Note at this point that the inner labia are the most tender spots. Using your tongue, make them flat and lick them, and then kiss them; using your tongue in a pointed fashion, make designs upon them.

Every woman has one very particular tender spot, and the touch of your tongue will make it feel especially sensitive. This is the spot that will bring her to orgasm. You do not yet know where that particular spot lies; it is up to you to discover this special area. There's no fun in asking where it is. Locate it yourself, and you will be amply rewarded for it. Once you find this spot, you will need to concentrate your efforts on it and remain there until her orgasm comes.

There are several spots on a woman that are rewarding. One is directly above the vaginal entrance, below the urethral opening. This spot is referred to as the U-spot, and in most women it brings great pleasure when you caress it with your tongue.

I suggest you place one or more pillows directly under her bottom, which will greatly aid in locating the U-spot easily with your mouth. Always make sure that you are as comfortable as you can be when you pleasure a woman with your tongue and mouth, as this is not a quick endeavor. There is a high probability that you will remain in the same position for a few minutes or perhaps even as long as several hours. And don't forget your hands! Place your two hands under her bottom. She will be more comfortable and feel a connection with you.

The area directly above the clitoral hood is another area where most women enjoy being licked. You will also want to try sucking the glans clitoris between your lips ever so gently. Now, for some women, this area is far too sensitive, and they cannot enjoy this. Pay close attention to her reactions. You may also try entering her vagina, moving your tongue in and out of her, as some women particularly love that. Remember that each woman is different, and no one particular movement pleases all.

At this stage of exploration, you need to be meticulously slow, and you must watch and listen to her body. You will feel her body begin to move up and down as well as shake. Much like a musical instrument, a vulva will vibrate and speak to you. If you have doubts, check whether she has indications of extreme sexual excitement.

Granted, every woman is unique in this regard: Perhaps this particular woman's nipples get hard when she's excited, or perhaps she's the kind who only has hardened nipples in the midst of orgasm. On the other hand, she may be the type who flushes red whenever she is excited, or else only during orgasm. Some women tremble a lot, and some "speak" to you with their feet.

Be thoroughly aware of her signals, and you will become a much more sensitive lover. You'll know you have found her magic spot when these signals appear. Some women will even tell you, "I am ready to have an orgasm, whenever you are ready I can give to you."

If the moment hasn't arrived yet, you may even try to feel her clitoris to see if it's gotten hard enough to peek out of its hood. If so, you may lick it, but even if it is not visually evident, consider that it may be waiting underneath. Use your tongue to investigate, going above the vulva and feeling for her clitoris. It may be difficult to find, but even if you cannot find that tiny pearl, you can still make it rise by licking the covering that hides it.

Lick harder now and press your tongue into the skin; with your fingers, carefully pull the labia away and extend your tongue to flick the clitoris, whether it is covered with the hood or not. Do it quickly. You should feel her legs shudder at this point. When you sense she's reached the stage closest to orgasm, make an O with your lips and pull the clitoris into your mouth. Begin to suck on it gently and look at her face for a reaction. If she's expressing pleasure, start sucking harder. If she loves it, do it even harder. If she expresses undue sensitivity or says she's not ready yet, back off.

If, on the other hand, she begins to lift her pelvis toward you due to the tension of the pending orgasm, stay with her every movement and do not pressure her otherwise. Whatever you do, keep it up, hang on, and maintain your mouth on her clitoris. She herself may well be saying, "Don't stop, whatever you do, don't stop!".

No matter what, even if you are painfully erect and were long ago ready to penetrate her, do not stop. Women are so angry when men stop there. They rant and rail that the man stopped. They feel that men never "get it," and they are totally frustrated.

Thus you must concentrate at this point and be thoroughly focused on her. The most common reason for failure of cunnilingus is that the male begins to think about work, about football, or about the time that could be spent otherwise. Concentration on what you are doing at this time is vital.

Most women feel an intensification of pleasure if you penetrate them at the same time that you perform oral stimulation. You can use two fingers or a vibrator. If you use two fingers, you will massage her G-spot at the same time, you may either massage her vagina toward you like a "come here" motion or opposite way. This way she mostly start to ejaculate on your face rapidly. She will be delighted and you too. My favorite technique, because it is easy is to push my two fingers right on the G-spot, keeping my finger still while I stimulate her orally. Another technique is to position your two fingers down her vagina toward her perinea. She will feel like she is been penetrated at the same time as been licked. Your chances of success may be better if you consider using a special G-spot vibrator like: Posh g-spot vibrator and Vibe Gigi G-spot . That may prove to be less tiring for you and actually bring even better results. Perhaps you will choose to continue the G-spot massage (see Chapter 7) even after she has had her orgasm—some women like that, and some do not. It depends how her vulva and clitoris become sensitive after her first orgasm. *(see pictures of vibrators: Posh g-spot vibrator and Vibe Gigi G-spot)*

Venus Butterfly Technique

For example, one woman once contacted me saying "*I am somewhat newly divorced after a very long term marriage. I consider myself a sexual person that is coming alive a little later in life. I usually come quickly, but would enjoy the process of some delay. I think I have had a G–spot orgasm, but I am not sure. Exploring that is also of interest to me.*" Once, I read it, I thought the Venus Butterfly technique would be perfect for her. The main thing is to keep your Goddess on plateau and delaying her orgasm as much as possible,

Some women are able to reach orgasm easily, whereas others need quite a lot of stimulation before they climax with pleasure. Always make your partner feel comfortable, and take your time to pleasure her. A woman can feel when her partner is in a hurry and getting frustrated that he is not able to make her come. It is most important to create an environment that is relaxed and open.

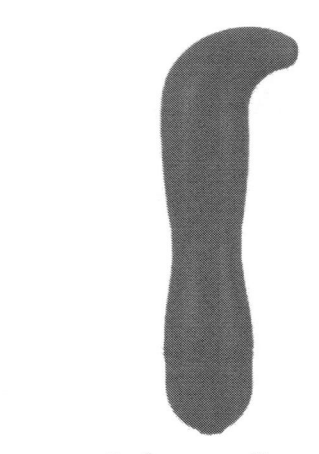

Posh g-spot vibrator

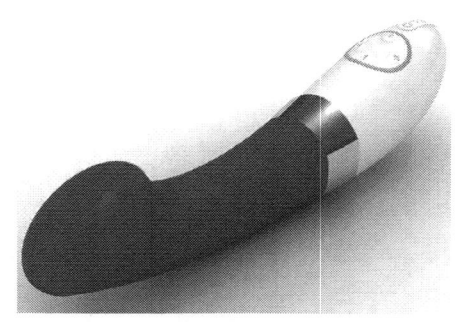

Vibe Gigi G-spot

By moving the stimulation between her clitoris and her vagina (like a butterfly returning to a flower again and again!), you can bring a woman to an ultimate orgasm. Stimulate your woman's clitoris, and as soon as you feel her ready to have an orgasm, stop and move your stimulation to the vagina for a few seconds. Gently go back to her clitoris, and stimulate this area again until she is about to come, then move on to pleasuring the rest of her vagina. Do this a few times, until you decide to let her having her pleasure. As soon as she reaches her orgasm, slip your finger(s) palm side up inside her vagina and tap the G-spot, which is approximately 2 inches inside, on the upper wall of the vagina, between the pubic bone and the cervix.

You can also use vibrator, or fingers to stimulate clitoris and vagina. However you choose to proceed, the idea is not to let her reach orgasm immediately, but to keep her on the edge as long as she can bear the teasing while stimulating her G-spot at the same time (Chapter 7 has more on this). All of this teasing and playing could even make her experience multiple orgasms.

Show Him You Love It

Ladies, remember that this man who is pleasuring you with cunnilingus is a jewel you have discovered. Tell him he is in the right spot. Put your hands on his head and push his head against your pelvis. This pressure against your vulva will accentuate your pleasure. Talk to him, and tell him when you are ready to have your orgasm, and then let yourself be free and release your sexual energy. Remember: in Tantra, everything is together; Tantra is a perfect union wherein sex becomes a sacrament of love. After you have been pleasured so much, tell him no one ever gave you so much pleasure. Tell him he is the God to your Goddess.

After the Fireworks, another Firework

Once a woman has had an orgasm, do not leave her in the throes of pleasure to seek your own pleasure or to sleep. She will prefer to enjoy the great connection you have, so talk to her, stroke her body, and caress her breasts. She may rest for a while, but because you've begun to awaken her, she may be ready for your best oral sex once more. This is the superlative means of making a woman multi orgasmic, so that you can both enjoy her forays into the ecstasy she is capable of.

Remember that males are totally different from females in this respect: A man can roll over and instantly fall asleep after his orgasm, feeling no sense of loss whatsoever, much less remorse. This is the result of the hormones prolactin, oxytocin, and vasopressin, which induce sleep after ejaculation, so don't blame the male too much for this. However, a woman's nature requires cuddling after sex.

Cunnilingus Exercise

Be sure to share this chapter with your partner and begin practicing today. Make him understand how important it is for you to have oral sex. If he is not used to oral sex, make it a fun experience for him. For instance, apply or pour chocolate, cream, jam, or Champagne on your vulva, and ask him to taste it. He will love the sweetness, forget his inhibitions, and start enjoying the game.

Motivational Moment

If you are a man and are going to take this chapter to heart, you will be heralded as a great lover. If you are a female and are sharing this chapter and its secrets, you will have a wonderful future sex life.

Stimulating the Vulva and Anus with Fingers

When it comes to making love, there are many ways to bring pleasure to your female partner besides penetration. One of these ways is via stimulation of the vulva and anus with your fingers. Let's be clear: Some women masturbate daily or even several times a day. They know exactly how to have an orgasm and how long it takes for them to reach that pleasure, but sometimes they crave a human touch. Satisfying this desire is the reason that you are in her bedroom tonight.

Unfortunately, many women worry that you will not be patient enough to give them an orgasm, based on previous experiences they have had with men who let them down. Be patient, and do not worry. You have the whole night to please her. Surprise her! Be a man with a lot of knowledge and many tender touches, and you will become her favorite lover.

Remember to have your nails cut, wash your hands, and use a water-based lubricant; better yet, wear gloves if you are going to stimulate her G-spot for a long time. I have met women who told me they were ready to seek medical attention the day after too much finger stimulation, concerned about their urethral pain.

Here are some techniques that will bring her multiple orgasms:

Clitoral Stimulation with Fingers

Please always remember that your fingers should never be dry when touching a woman's vulva. Keep them wet by using a gel enhancer or water-based lube (or some saliva). Do not treat the stimulation of the clitoris as foreplay, but make it your main course.

Little Orgasmic Secrets

A woman who does not have or rarely has orgasms with her partner is not going to tell you; she is going to fake it, always. My survey shows that 75 percent of women have faked orgasm at least one or more times, and that 45 percent experience limited sexual pleasure with their partners, even if a woman happens to be very orgasmic when she undertakes self-pleasure. (Go to www.mysecretquiz.com, and you can take the quiz too!) Most women keep hoping that one day she will meet a man who will know how to satisfy her with the ultimate sexual pleasure. It could be you and her search could stop right here because you learn how to satisfy your Goddess , and to make her come first.

In some situations, sexual enhancers can be very helpful for clitoral stimulation. These products for women (completely different from a lube like K-Y Jelly) stimulate her mentally and increase vaginal blood flow and lubrication in her vagina, with the result that the G-spot then becomes more engorged. Enhancers also increase the blood flow to the clitoris, making her more sensitive to stimulation and also allowing her to have better and more orgasms.

Even if you are good at pleasing your Goddess, there is no harm in asking her which ways give her the most pleasure when she masturbates. Most women will be more than happy to show them to you by masturbating in front of you. You will learn a lot by watching your partner masturbate. You will find out her most sensitive point(s) and be able to repeat her movements.

Ask your partner to lie on her back with her knees bent and her legs spread, in order to expose her yoni to you. This way you can see her clitoris, and her excitation will increase if she likes being watched.

Prior to engaging in a finger stimulation massage in the clitoris area, you should first massage her legs, thighs, and abdomen, and then touch the labia with your palm to prepare your Goddess for the stimulation of the clitoris. With your left hand, gently spread her labia, and with your right hand, start to tease her clitoral area.

Your fingers should always be as light and soft as possible, and your touch should feel like a feather. Be very gentle, and go very slowly.

Different techniques

- From the hood, pinch gently and press up and down on her clitoris (*see drawing: From the hood, pinch gently and press up and down her clitoris*)

- Rub in circular motion and pressing at the same time on the hood of her clitoris with your fingers or the palm of your hand. The motion may start slowly then faster and faster when she is ready to reach her orgasm. Many women masturbate that way.

- Take her vulva between your two fingers and gently press up and down with her vulva against each other and release and press again, until you feel her orgasm.

- Most women have a very special point at 1 o'clock or (but less often) at 11o'clock from her clitoris. It is either left or right from her clitoris. Very gently find that point with the tip of your finger. You will feel it - listen to her body, she will tell you, "yes right there", then rub and don't stop until she reaches her orgasm.

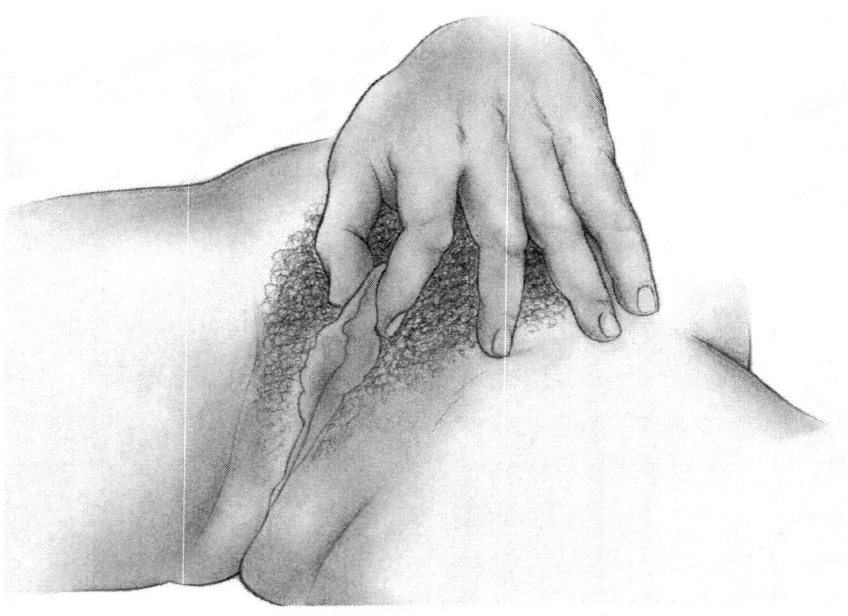

From the hood, pinch gently and press up and down her clitoris

Once, a woman has her first orgasm, the clitoris becomes very sensitive. She needs rest, take her in your arms and make her feel closer to your heart. She will deeply appreciate that intimacy. Some women who are very orgasmic will not need rest after her first orgasm and wish that you carry on without interruption.

Vaginal Stimulation with Fingers

The insertion of a finger into the vagina (or the anus) should be done with care and patience. Let the motion of the muscles of her orifice absorb and attract your finger inside of her. Do not push your finger against her muscles as it may hurt her. Both orifices have strong muscles that slowly take your finger in. It is much more erotic for a woman to want you and to attract you inside of her than to be rushed into anything.

After stimulating her clitoris, insert your middle finger in her vagina, gently exploring her inside. When she is wet enough, you can gradually insert more fingers. Most men only use an in-and-out motion with their fingers, as they do during intercourse, but women are more aroused by a circular motion with varied depth and speed. This way you stroke all the walls of her vagina, increasing the excitation.

Use your finger (one or two) to stroke and rub the anterior wall of the vagina, as you would do in a "come here" gesture. You should feel a portion of spongy tissue; this is the G-spot. Remember that the G-spot is easy to feel under stimulation. The G-spot is situated opposite the clitoris, in the upper wall of the vagina.

Use double stimulation: While your index and middle finger stimulate her G-spot, use your thumb (or tongue) to gently rub her clitoris. Then slowly, you may accelerate your motion as long and fast you can as if you were simulating a penis penetration. She will moan saying *"OMG what are you doing to me"* and twist her body with pleasure and most probably have an orgasm. This is one of the most powerful finger stimulation techniques, a rewarding one that a man should master.

Anal Stimulation with Fingers

Dear Jean-Claude, I have had two partners in the recent past that awakened my interest in anal pleasure. Both were gentle in their approach and I found the experience pleasurable. Once, on one occasion my partner used plenty of lubricant and slowly introduced one finger and then another and possibly a third, I don't recall exactly as I was giving him oral stimulation as he was fingering my anus. He was able to bring me to orgasm and G-spot orgasm via my anus and it was a very good feeling that I enjoyed. On another occasion, the same partner brought me to a G-spot orgasm by anal penetration and simultaneous vaginal finger stimulation.

A different partner was able to elicit a squirting orgasm by penetrating my anus with his fingers and was able to insert his entire hand in my vagina simultaneously and when he pulled out his hand and all the fluid came out, I had the longest and most full body "orgasm" I have ever experienced. Karen S.

Ask your partner to lie face down, with her legs slightly apart and knees bent. This position will not only facilitate your access to her anus, but also expose her yoni for massage. (*see drawing: This position will not only facilitate your access to her anus, but also expose her yoni for massage*)

Prior to anal stimulation with fingers, the area should be stimulated with lots of licking. See paragraph about Analingus. Massage the buttocks using a circular motion, then slide your hand along her buttocks to her inner thigh and labia. Spread her buttocks with your left hand, and then slide your wet finger between the buttocks, brushing the anus. Stimulate the anus using gentle strokes and circular rubbing until your partner starts moving her hips up and down, allowing you to enter the anus.

Use your pinky or your middle finger to penetrate the anus very slowly (be sure it is well lubricated), and stimulate it from the inside, using in-and-out motions as well as circular ones. Often, a Goddess is very responsive to having her anus fingered gently and slowly and at the same time feeling your finger massaging her G-spot through the thin wall of the anus. It is important to know, that the excitement of the anal finger stimulation is not in an in and out motion only, but more in the massage a anal cavity for your finger to be able to massage the vagina area or G-spot through the very thin wall between the two cavities. A great anal stimulation could easily result of incredible clitoral or vaginal orgasm and female ejaculation.

Use triple stimulation: For this, your pinkie stimulates the anus, your index and middle finger stimulate the vagina and her G-spot, and your thumb rubs her clitoris. This is a Tantric technique called "To Hold One of World's Greatest Mysteries in Your Hand." Your partner will experience a pleasure she has never felt before and could even come to orgasm multiple times. (Wash your hands if you intend to stimulate her vagina after this).

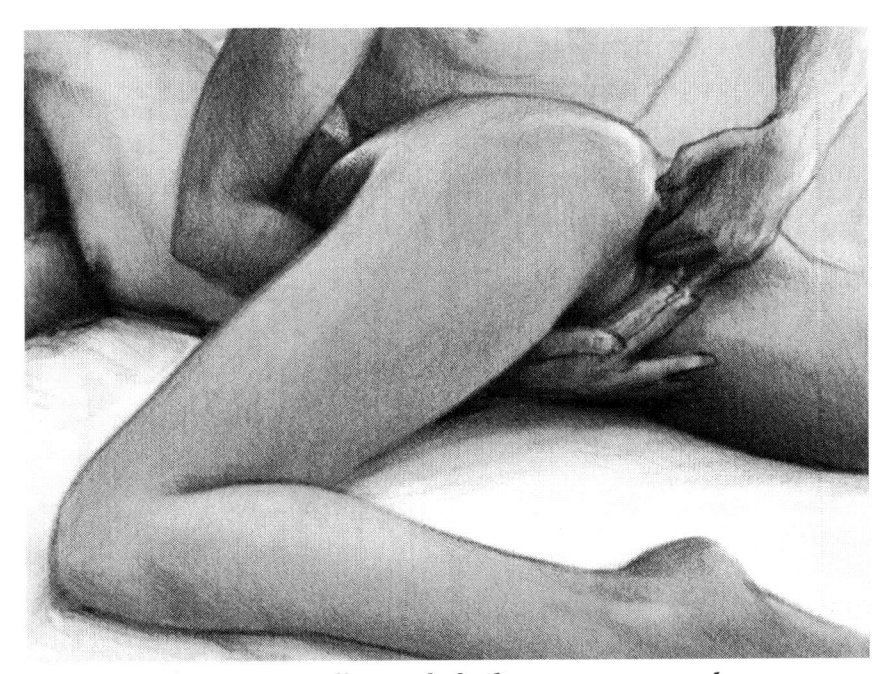

This position will not only facilitate your access to her anus, but also expose her yoni for massage

Sometimes for a woman, it is easier to have an orgasm with vaginal penetration (or simultaneous anal and vaginal penetration) while having the clitoris stimulated at the same time. I know this is not easy to do if you do not have experience. I often use a vibrator in each orifice, and that way it is easy for me to focus on stimulating her vulva. The secret is to gradually prepare her for multiple orgasms and not go straight for the clitoris. After you master the basic techniques, resulting in a positive sexual adventure for both of you, variations of different techniques are encouraged.

Analingus followed by fingers stimulation of the anal area are the first steps prior to a successful anal intercourse. Be as gentle with your penis as you are with your finger, slowly and gentle, plenty of lube is the key to enjoy anal sex. Anal penetration is often reported by women as a full body experience if prior to that practice, most of the erogenous zones have been explored and stimulated. A woman emailed me, saying *"I am so attracted by anal sex but the last guy who tried was so rough that I have been discouraged for long time. I would like to know if there is a way to make that pleasure less painful?"*

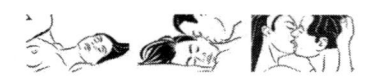

Exercise for Vulval and Anal Stimulation

Use Tantric massage to arouse your partner; then ask her to masturbate in front of you. If she does not want to touch herself in front of you, put your fingers on her clitoris and ask her to put her hand over yours and guide your motions. Do not oppose her rhythm or direction; follow her guidance and allow her to feel the pleasure. The next time, try to recreate the rhythm and motions she showed you, adding some of your own, and see what she likes.

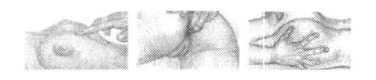

Motivational Moment

If you want to impress your female lover and help her reach a new level of pleasure, consider reserving some time to stimulate her yoni with tenderness and dedication. By learning how to stimulate the yoni and the anus at the same time, your partner will experience an orgasm twice as powerful as a normal one, and her orgasms will grow in intensity if you continue the stimulation.

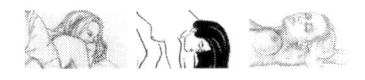

Note about Analingus, Cunnilingus and Finger Stimulation

This chapter addressed the taboo of analingus, why it is so very exciting and pleasurable, and how analingus can be utilized to bring you to greater heights of pleasure.

In this chapter you also learned that the vulva is a precious jewel, and that cunnilingus is a very precise but easy technique. You learned how to make the experience enjoyable and successful, so that you and your partner will love it.

In the end, this chapter opened the gate to a whole different realm of providing pleasure for your partner. You learned how to help her relax, how to use your fingers to stimulate her vulva, and how to use techniques that will maximize the pleasure she will experience.

Fill in this log to record the results of your exercises:

1. Which pleasurable taboos did you explore this week: Ask your partner to do analingus, cunnilingus, or a G-spot massage? Use chocolate cream, jam, Champagne?

2. What change do you want to see in yourself spiritually and sexually?

3. How do you feel about your own sexuality, now that you have done these exercises?

4. On a scale of 1 to 10, with 10 the maximum, how have these exercises improved the quality of your orgasm(s)?

	1	2	3	4
Week 1				
Week 2				
Week 3				
Week 4				
Week 5				
Week 6				
Week 7				
Week 8				

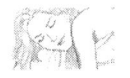

CHAPTER 6

Self-Pleasure or Masturbation

It was Valentine's Day, and I was going to spend it alone—or so I imagined. On this day, many women set out to be pampered and loved by their boyfriends and husbands and in turn take these men to bed, only to be let down after a great evening. Men too often focus on what they believe a woman's needs are, not on what the particular woman actually needs.

That evening someone called me. "You told me you were a coach and Tantric masseur, and gave me your business card the other day when were waiting in the cell phone shop."

"Yes, I remember. You were wearing a Balsa Wood perfume. Omnia from Bvlgari? I love that fragrance. It brings me back so beautiful memories"

"Yes, exactly. You are good! I'm Melanie. I am a screenwriter, like many of us in the city of stars. I am house-sitting in the San Fernando Valley at the moment. I have been through some very traumatic and nightmarish times in my life, especially in the last two years."

"My husband died in a very bad work accident two and a half years ago. This has resulted in me feeling that parts of me are scattered and horribly diminished. I feel on some level that perhaps you can help me. It *seems I cannot show love and affection to the men I truly care about, or even to myself."*

"I am in a strange place. This is, undoubtedly, affecting my entire life, and I am at loss to know what to do to turn this all around. I've gained a lot of weight. Others tell me I look great, but I know what I used to look like. I met a man I started seeing a few weeks ago. There is a spark missing that I know he cannot fill; it is missing within myself. But I notice he is trying to mold me into his perfect woman. That bothers me. He also lost his wife a year ago due to a hospital error. I have not been very orgasmic for many years. I am thinking your coaching would be good for me."

"I looked at the subjects you coach women in, and they are all very wonderful. But most of all, I would like you to teach me how to pleasure myself. It seems very stupid, probably, but believe me, I have never done it. I had a very strict upbringing. My father was in the military, and it was not the kind of subject I would dare talk about around the dinner table."

I was soon out the door, heading down the Interstate toward the San Fernando Valley. Traffic was busy, as usual. Everyone was on their way to their dates, looking for love and affection. I, however, was on my way to coach a beautiful woman to help her understand that there is nothing wrong with her features, and that self-pleasure is the basis of discovering and enjoying her body. It is certainly one of the safest sexual acts, and the least disappointing!

Melanie was beautiful: deep golden-brown skin the color of toasted sesame seeds and, sprinkled with cinnamon freckles; tightly curled ringlets of hair, the color of black coffee. Her mouth was wide, with full lips and a ready smile, but her eyes told a different story.

A few days after our meeting, she wrote in our correspondence that the meeting between us was a gift to herself at a time in her life when she had little to be grateful for. She told me, "When you walked through my door,

I was met with some of the most inconceivably loving eyes, energy, and presence. I knew I had made the right decision. Your French parents did an incredible job of raising you, and I just want to thank them. I want to thank you for opening a door to what now what will be a difficult but rewarding journey."

In the modern world, self-pleasure is no longer a taboo topic. Female self-pleasure is that small, intimate joy that eliminates stress and fatigue. It contributes to the mental and emotional relaxation every woman deserves to feel.

The reasons why you should experience self-pleasure are several:

- Self-pleasure offers a suitable way for a woman to connect with herself. Self-pleasure is practically a rite of transformation of sexual energy into spiritual energy, with the sole purpose of providing pleasure.

- Orgasm or ejaculation is not the only goal of self-pleasure. When a woman expresses her love for herself–for her body and for her personality–this increases her confidence, attractiveness, and knowledge of herself and her magnetism.

- Self-pleasure provides an opportunity for women to know their own bodies, and if they wish, they can reach an orgasm. Like any skill, self-pleasure requires experience, guarding against injury, and enough time for quiet study of the body.

Erroneous Perceptions of Female Self-Pleasure

Self-pleasure does not make women the enemy of sex with a partner; on the contrary, it adds to their sex life. It is wrong to think that if a woman has a steady partner, she does not need self-pleasure or that there is a problem in the couple's sex life.

Many married women have told me, "I love my husband, and I love to have sex with him, but self-pleasure gives me a different satisfaction. I need to do it because it makes me feel self-confident and definitely more attractive. Many men eye me now. I even notice that since I found the secret of self-pleasure, my self-esteem has increased, and I began to love myself more. It is also reflected in those closest to me, because now I give them more love too."

Men, make no mistake, masturbate as much as women. There is no reason for women or men to feel ill-treated or insecure about a form of sexual release that a partner can perform on him or herself. This is a part of the pleasure that our bodies can offer us, and masturbation can teach us many useful things about sex with a partner.

Ideas on How and Where to Provide Yourself Pleasure

1. You can decide by yourself where to provide self-pleasure. The first thing to do is to secure a peaceful place where you feel comfortable.

2. You can dim your bedroom lights, light a few scented candles, and put satin sheets on the bed where you will indulge.

3. You can do it in your garden or somewhere private you are directly in connection with our nature: trees, plants, sky and sun.

4. You can fill your bathtub with aromatic salts and relax to the maximum in the warm water.

5. At this point, your goal is to connect with yourself, to stay only with you—*your* thoughts and *your* feelings. It is important to relax and open your soul to the feelings you hide in your most secret recesses, whatever they may be: love, joy, hatred, or anger.

6. Do not let thoughts of everyday problems worry you at this time. If the bathtub is the place you feel comfortable and peaceful, then you can start the self-pleasure there. You can begin by stroking different parts of your body: face, neck, arms, abdomen, legs, and feet. Then you will feel the desire to go to the erogenous zones: breasts, vagina, and anus. Explore your body through slow, flowing movements of your hands and fingers, and don't go rushing to your clitoris. The aim is to awaken your sexual energy and redirect it to other parts of your body—and to your heart and mind. Enjoy every touch of your skin!

7. Close your eyes and imagine times you felt loved, attractive, and irresistible. Let these feelings possess you, so that you can better connect with yourself.

8. The time it will take to self-pleasure depends only on you. At some point, you will feel the need to start light and smooth movements on your clitoris, and eventually these will quicken. Do it! To save the emerging power within you just before an orgasm occurs, however, stop caressing your clitoris and relax. You will feel a strong wave of energy that circulates through your body and spreads to all of its parts. This is the ultimate moment in self-pleasure, when each cell in your body is excited and loaded with energy.

9. Of course, if you wish, you can reach orgasm. If your body shivers, your nipples harden, the areolas of your breasts darken, your face reddens, and your clitoris becomes so sensitive that you can no longer touch it, then you are in a state of orgasm.

10. Feel free to relax and enjoy the excitement, but know that after several minutes you can get another orgasm by touching your

clitoris with your fingers, by squeezing your thighs, or by using an object to stimulate the clitoris.

Finding Your Clitoris

Putting direct pressure and making circular movements on the glans or head of the clitoris and along the shaft and crura or "forks" of the clitoris will produce sexual arousal. While stroking the clitoris, you can also place a finger in direct contact with the clitoral skin, moving the entire clitoral glans around beneath the surface, sliding and tugging it upward against its hood or covering.

In the same way that a man strokes the corona of his penis in a capping and twisting motion during masturbation, the idea is to stroke the corona of the glans of the clit rather than the top of the glans directly. Stroking along the crura just off-center from the top of the glans also produces an extreme state of arousal. This is similar to the effect produced in a man by stroking the frenulum of the penis and below the penile glans.

For some, rubbing the foreskin or hood of the clitoris is not pleasurable; instead, if the foreskin is first gently pushed away from the glans before stroking it in a circular motion, then sexual arousal is enhanced. Exposing the glans first in this way is the equivalent of a man pulling his foreskin down and away from the glans as the penis becomes erect when he masturbates.

Once the clitoris is erect and the glans exposed, stroking along the crura of the clitoral shaft in an upward stroke produces intense pleasure. In the same way, many men experience ultimate pleasure when their penis is stroked in an upward motion from root to tip during masturbation and intercourse. To perfect the upward motion, it is important to understand that the clitoral shaft branches into two crura that extend on each side of the clitoral glans. The direction of the circular stroke will determine which portion of the movement is upward and which portion is downward. When moving your finger in a clockwise manner around the clitoral glans, the upward movement is from 9 o'clock' to noon on the "clock." The 11 o'clock position is generally regarded as the most arousing spot on the clitoral crura, and by pressing this point in a firm but gentle manner; some women experience the sensation of orgasm without contraction or culmination.

It is important to understand that each person is different, and so the location that produces the greatest sensations of sexual intensity will vary from person to person. Take the time to explore your body and learn which type of stimulation arouses you the most. Then, be open to sharing this knowledge with your partner.

Finding Your G-Spot

While you are self-pleasuring, it is a good idea to try to locate your G-spot. This part of the vaginal wall has a slightly different texture than the surrounding tissue and is rough to the touch. When you probe, you can easily locate the island of the G-spot because the contrast between it and the surrounding tissue is very significant. Some women appreciate experiencing G-spot pleasure without depending on a partner.

- This zone is very sensitive, with high concentrations of nerve receptors. Its main function is the ultimate sexual pleasure sensation.

- Absolutely every woman has a G-spot, but in different representatives of the fair sex it may vary in both size and placement.

- According to some women, stimulation of the G-spot leads to deeper and broader pleasure than stimulation of the clitoris!

The most common location for the G-spot is in the front wall of the vagina, but do remember that variations are possible. If you do not find your G-spot immediately, do not worry but search to the side or back. Sometimes the G-spot can be in a different location at the side or in the back near the rear vaginal wall.

1. Explore with your finger, using a mirror to find the vaginal opening. (Some ladies are unable to orient themselves to the "right hole".)

2. You may sit, but it's better to lie flat on your back.

3. Spread your feet as wide apart as possible for better access to your vagina.

4. With palms facing upward toward your belly, drag one or two fingers until their tops rest against the anterior vaginal wall or squeeze the upper wall of the vagina.

5. Slide your fingers from the entranceway very slowly! If they do not drag/slide, use slight pressure to allow your fingertips to explore your vagina gently. When you reach a place where the tissue is slightly different in composition than its surroundings, you have reached your G-spot. With your fingers curled in a "come hither" motion you want to pull out your fingers from your vagina. Many women prefer to explore their G-spot by themselves. With patience and passion you will be able to have a female ejaculation. You will be very exited and overwhelmed to reach that level of pleasure.

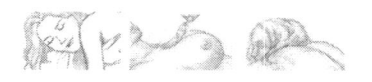

Exercises for Self-Pleasure Using Fingers and/or Vibrator

It is time to proceed to the erogenous zone of your clitoris. Your fingers are ideal tools to learn what kind of pressure, velocity, and movement do the best job for you. The indisputable advantage of this type of sex is that you are the sovereign mistress of the situation.

The Figure 8 is a good place to start. When fingers (one or more), glide around the clitoris, making the shape of an 8, they stimulate the labia minora. Since the lips have many nerve endings, touching them brings women more excitement and pleasure than straight clitoral stimulation. Many women have shared that this pleasure really is bigger. Here's how to try it:

1. Using your forefinger and middle finger, drag them east-west and north-south over your most sensitive area.

2. With your forefinger and ring finger, open the lips and move the middle finger on the central section. Enjoy these signs of excitement: rapid breathing, ruffled hair, and blood pulsing in your veins.

3. Do not forget to stimulate other parts of your body with your free hand for full delight.

4. The finish line can be reached by inserting one or more fingers in your vagina, imitating the penetration of a penis.

When it comes to sex and self-pleasure, vibrators are great tools, providing one of the strongest forms of erotic stimulation.

Using a sex toy is matter of choice. Some women love toys, and others would rather use their fingers. If you are tempted to use a toy, it is time to go online, or else lose your fear of entering the sex shop in your town and ask there for some advice. The choice is very large these days. I met a lady who uses her Sybian sex machine daily because her husband, who is many years older than she, cannot satisfy her any more. (see *picture of vibrator Sybian*)

Some suggestions for using your vibrator: (see *picture of vibrator Jelly Vibrator*)

1. Start by sliding the toy over your panties, allowing the vibrations to gradually move and spread in your body.
2. Next, proceed to direct contact.
3. For maximum rise in tension, put off increasing speed.
4. If you experience tingling and numbness of the area, do not worry; this is a temporary reaction. Simply carry on with other sensual areas for a few minutes.

You can easily provide yourself a double pleasure by using a vibrator designed for the G-spot (which is bent at the end) and your fingers. With the vibrator you will reach your G-spot, and with your fingers you will stimulate your clitoris. When you feel comfortable with your body and ready to explore more, you may find it helpful to read the section in Chapter 7 about self-pleasuring of the G-spot.

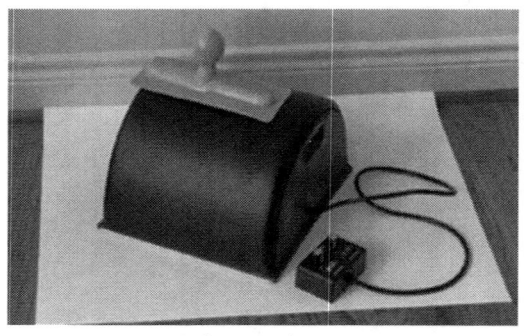

Sybian Vibrator

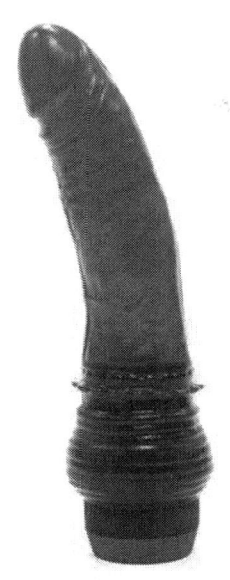

Jelly Vibrator

Types of Vibrators

Realistic Vibrator: A copy of the penis. Since it can bend, it allows you to stimulate your G-spot. In addition, you can use it for external stimulation of the clitoris. (*see pictures: double stimulation dildo and penis and clitoris vibrator*)

Simultaneous G-spot/Clitoris Vibrator: This type of vibrator uses a vibrating tip for intense stimulation of the clitoris from your vagina. (*see picture of the vibrator Butterfly Kiss*)

Double-Stimulation Vibrator: Features a swivel head that can vibrate and pulsate at different speeds, allowing you to choose the degree of pleasure you want. (*see picture double stimulation dildo*)

148   Sex: Woman First

Vibrator Warning

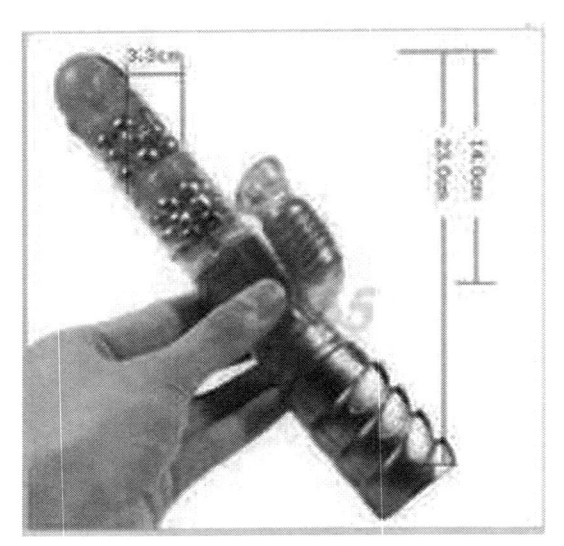

Double stimulation dildo and penis

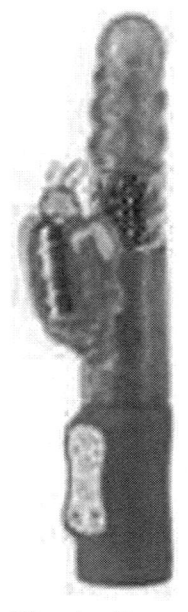

Clitoris vibrator

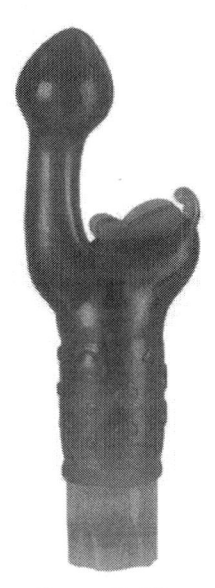

Butterfly Kiss

Using a vibrating device (massager or vibrator) too frequently may desensitize the clitoris as intense stimulation of the G-spot and urethral nerves may trigger the release of collagen protein. This hardens the clitoral and G-spot erectile tissues, leading to poor clitoral, vulval, and vaginal blood circulation—and ultimately, to sexual and orgasmic dysfunction, or female impotency.

Abuse of masturbation with a vibrator may erode the clitoral tissue, which will lead to low libido, sexual arousal disorder, and orgasmic dysfunction.

You should also be cautious that you do not become dependent on a high-speed vibrator to achieve your best orgasms, thereby becoming independent of your partner. You should instead educate your partner, explaining what you want and need instead of relying always on the vibrator to deliver. This is my personal opinion, with the aim of ensuring that you do not endanger your relationship. For some women, private pleasure may be more important; this is a personal choice.

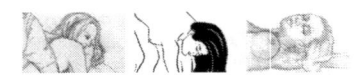

Motivational Moment

Any woman who loves and respects herself can self-pleasure and receive maximum positive benefits:

- Self-pleasure relieves stress and tension and loads the body with energy.
- Orgasm strengthens the immune system and pelvic floor muscles.
- Self-pleasure can help you maintain better relationships through the production of oxytocin, a hormone related to social skills and personality.
- Self-pleasure offers you a way to satisfy yourself whenever you want and as often you like.
- Self-pleasure helps you to understand where and how you want to be touched, so that you'll feel content.
- Self-pleasure helps relieve depressive emotions and keeps you in a good mood.
- Self-pleasure increases your self-knowledge and deepens your relationship with yourself.
- Self-pleasure strengthens your relationship with your partner.

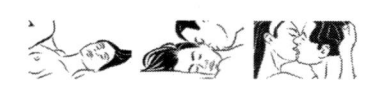

Note about Self-Pleasure

Self-pleasure is a privilege for every woman. In this chapter you found out why some women choose self-pleasure, whether they are alone or in a relationship. You learned where and how you can provide yourself with unmatched satisfaction and which areas you need to pay attention to. A sense of self-control when interacting with your body, mind, and soul brings unique spiritual and sexual satisfaction, the combination of which gives rise to the ultimate female pleasure.

Fill in this log to record the results of your exercises:

1. Did you experience self-pleasure this week: Did you explore your anatomy (yoni, the crown jewel, vagina, breasts, G-spot)? Did you practice self-pleasure with fingers? A vibrator?

2. What change do you want to see in yourself spiritually and sexually?

3. How do you feel about your own sexuality, now that you have done these exercises?

4. On a scale of 1 to 10, with 10 the maximum, how have these exercises improved the quality of your orgasm(s)?

	1	2	3	4
Week 1				
Week 2				
Week 3				
Week 4				
Week 5				
Week 6				
Week 7				
Week 8				

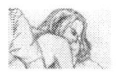

CHAPTER 7

Exploring the A-spot and the G-spot

The A-spot and Its Pleasures

The A-spot, formally called the anterior fornix erogenous zone (AFE zone), is my preferred spot in a woman. It is hidden as though it where a nice little secret, but at the same time, it is fairly easy to find and gives a woman one of the greatest sexual pleasures. The A-spot is truly a diamond in the rough and has serious importance in the erotic massage of a woman.

The Malaysian sex scientist Dr. Chua Chee Ann, discovered the A-spot. In the midst of his research with female subjects suffering from vaginal dryness, he found that stimulation of an area deep in the vagina on the anterior wall resulted in rapid lubrication and arousal. (It is interesting that he did not make his discovery public until thirteen years after he made it. Who knows—maybe he was so astonished that he wanted to keep his little secret for himself! If you're interested in following up, here's what he has said about his discovery: http://www.aspot-pioneer.com/pdf/DrChuaInterviewScript.pdf

Location

The A-spot is located about 3 1/2 to 4 inches inside the vagina, and it has a smooth feel. Unlike the G-spot, which (as discussed in Chapter 6) is located on the front wall of the vagina, the A-Spot is sensitive all the way around the circumference of the vagina. Massage of the A-spot should be handled very delicately.

Medically, the word *anterior* refers to something that is "in front," and sure enough, the A-spot is in front of and above the cervix, at the innermost point of the vagina. The fancy scientific name also refers to the recess or alcove that the upper (superior) segment of the woman's vagina forms above the cervix. This is called the fornix (*please see drawing: Scientists increasingly call the Skene's glands the "female prostate" because they make secretions that are almost identical to the seminal fluid produced by the male prostate in chapter 7*). This recess or alcove is separated into four distinct portions: the anterior and posterior fornices and two portions at the sides known as the lateral fornices. The anterior fornix is laden with nerve endings and thus is highly erogenous. For simplicity's sake, "A" is for anterior—therefore, we call this sensitive area the A-spot.

The A-spot Response

This erogenous zone does a number of interesting things. For instance, stimulating it causes the vaginal muscles to contract, which always feels good! In addition, it also has the effect of creating instant vaginal lubrication, which we all know greatly aids in helping to induce orgasm, and an anal-orifice contraction during the orgasm.

Following Dr. Chua's discovery, AFE vibrators were invented specifically for the purpose of stimulating the A-spot. These long, thin devices are specially constructed so that their ends curve upward to properly probe this zone. (*see picture of AFE vibrators*)

The majority of the time, you should begin to touch an erogenous zone with a very gentle touch, but the A-spot calls for the application of a bit of pressure, massage in circle. Time is of extreme importance here as well; this area should be stimulated for approximately 5 to 10 minutes, but sometimes more time is needed, so just be patient.

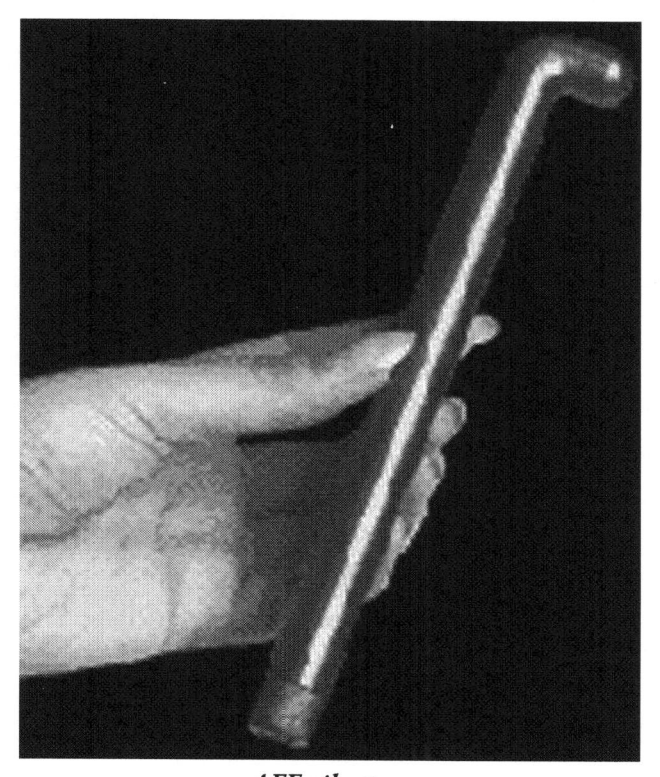

AFE vibrators

You do not need to stimulate the A-spot continuously until you get the desired effect. Instead, do a little bit every day. This will bring better results than stimulating for a long period of time in a desperate attempt to get results the first time. Chances are, you may not get any results the first time anyway, since your partner simply may not be ready mentally, spiritually, and physically.

Comfort Zone

Even if your lover isn't comfortable telling you what she wants, where she wants it, and for how long, the two of you have to be close enough and open enough to offer important feedback and encouragement. A-spot orgasms are patently dissimilar from other orgasms; thus it's an excellent idea to let your partner understand just how different this experience might be. The more you can prepare her, the more comfortable and relaxed she will be to begin her journey into the realm of the unknown.

The first thing you should suggest to your lover is that she attempt to pee. Some of the sensations caused by A-spot stimulation will make her suddenly feel like she has to urinate. This is because the A-spot is located very close to the bladder (*see drawing: Scientists increasingly call the Skene's glands the "female prostate" because they make secretions that are almost identical to the seminal fluid produced by the male prostate in chapter 7*). By going ahead and using the bathroom before heading into the bedroom, you'll prevent her from worrying about peeing.

If your lover does feels the desire to pee during A-spot stimulation, tell her it is okay. Tell her to let go. Of course, an incredible trust between the two of you is required for her to feel she can let go in that way and allow you to bring her to another level of sexuality. It is not a small thing, so be sure and thank her for her trust. In reality she won't pee but is only experiencing the sensation, which she will forget about after a while.

Positioning

Gentlemen, in order to find the A-spot best, you will want your lady to be on her back with her knees parted and bent so that you can easily enter her with your hand. You will be using your middle and index fingers. A woman will have a tremendously difficult time touching the A-spot herself. She cannot easily stimulate her A-spot with her own hands, and most likely your penis won't reach it either, unless it is very long. Remember that the A-spot is also called the "Deep Spot," and that's why it is ordinarily touched only by a partner's hands.

A partner can enter the vagina with an extended middle finger, or if he wishes, he may use two fingers, palm side up. Be sure and use plenty of lubrication such as K-Y Jelly or other. As with everything else in Tantric massage, this needs to be performed very slowly, letting the excitement of her vagina set your finger in motion along the vaginal wall.

Approximately 3 to 4 inches in, you will feel the rim of the anterior fornix, or A-spot. You will note that it is smooth and basically feels much like a Frisbee's rim. The cervix is located directly in the center and you will find that it resembles the tip of your nose. The cervix is, of course, the access to the uterus where babies are formed. Whether she likes her cervix to be touched or not differs greatly with each woman. Some women like to find the stimulation of the cervix very arousing. Always be gentle and adventurous.

Eventually, you will touch the A-zone. When you do, your fingers will be bathed in instant lubrication, enabling you to remember where you found the A-spot. Massage of the A-spot alone will not bring female ejaculation, but the pleasure is intense. Massage of the A-spot and the G-spot together will bring even greater pleasure and the possibility of female ejaculation. Generalities do not apply in matters of erogenous areas, but exploration and discovery of your particular woman's pleasure should be a great adventure.

In summary, here is the technique for A-spot massage:

1. Men at the beginning should stimulate the A-spot only by massaging in circles and then tapping against the vaginal wall.

2. After a bit, you will subsequently move your one or two fingers, depending on how comfortable you feel, in a circular manner all around the cervix.

3. You will note the color of your partner's face changing, and she will begin to moan loudly. Do not stop, you are in the right area for her to experience her first vaginal orgasm—although again, I caution you to not expect instant results!

4. When this first vaginal orgasm occurs, do not stop even then, but keep stimulating the area. Your lady should apply the breathing exercise mentioned in the second chapter. It is very important at this point to help her relax her mind and the PC (pubococcygeus) muscle. Encourage her to breathe together in synchronization with you, which will help you to build a bond by sharing this wonderful sexual experience.

A-Spot Exercise

Ladies, for your exercise today, I recommend that you purchase one of the long, thin, curved AFE vibrators and begin to play with it. Massage and stimulate your A-spot. After a while, you are going to find the right way to have an orgasm through this stimulation.

In some ways, I find it is important that you start to stimulate your A-spot yourself. I feel that overstimulation by your partner could bring forth disappointment. You see, the stimulation of any vaginal spot with the aim of producing an orgasm takes time and is not instantly rewarding. At times, my explanations may seem to be quite simple and easy, but there is also a large psychological element that can bring success or disappointment to any of these experiences. Women's sexuality is something very delicate; it all depends on how much a woman is ready to open up.

Once you have experienced its sensations and understand that your A-spot gives you great pleasure, you can then share the great news with your partner by saying, "Honey, I found something incredible when I pushed my vibrator deep inside me. It makes me feel absolutely wonderful, but I would much rather you do it with your long, beautiful finger."

Motivational Moment

As a man, I have sometimes been extremely surprised at the sensitivity of the A-spot, since it is far more sensitive than the G-spot. Its stimulation has brought me some great joy through the years, and my partners were always very thankful for it.

You can never learn too much about women. Consider what it will be like to be so skilled sexually that you can have a woman scream with untold pleasure, and you do all of this as though you'd done it all of your adult life? This is going to be a great tool! Massage the A-spot slowly and gently, and do not expect any results the first time. Just wait until she says, "Wow, it feels great! What did you do? Can you do it again?".

As a female, knowledge of this special area will ready you for your partner's help and enable you to have mind-shattering orgasms.

The Famous G-spot

I received her call early on a Saturday morning. Brianna told me that her psychotherapist had given her my business card. After two years of consulta-

tions, her therapist thought that she should try G-spot massage, which had changed the lives of some other clients. "She thinks you are a great person and I can trust you," Brianna explained. "The only day I'm available is Saturday," she added, with a very light Hispanic accent "I am thirty-four, and I work and go to school full time."

I explained briefly that, in general, women contact me because they need to feel more secure before dating again, or to explore their inner sexuality more deeply. Some want to feel their G-spot, be sure that they have one, and learn how to ejaculate or have multiple orgasms. All of these take time, but the results shouldn't take too long.

She replied, "I am heterosexual, and I have a variety of reasons why Tantric massage could help me. I'm ashamed of myself. When I was teenager, I used to have orgasms with my stepdad. He started off tickling and wrestling with me while gently touching me all over. The next thing I knew, he was rubbing my clit and pulling my panties off. I would help find ways for us to have our time alone. My stepdad and I played for about six months. Too many times my mom almost caught us.

"I have never played with myself, and I'm kind of shy, so it's hard for me to be open in my sexual life," Brianna went on. "I have thought that one of the reasons I'm like this is because I don't know my body's sensuality. I feel I don't have a lot of sensitivity on my breasts. It's very hard for me to be open with a man."

"Someone like you, who knows what you're doing, with the experience that you have—you could help me release all of these sexual traumas that I feel I've been carrying for so long. Today, I feel so lost sexually. Usually after I have sex with a man, I feel he is like a stranger and have no more attraction to him. All I want is to begin a healthy sexual life. I have heard that G-spot massage can do this for a woman," she concluded.

I replied, "Yes, you are right. You understood very well."

Not long after that, I was pulling up in front of her humble home, which she shared with friends. Outside, the cold-season winds were blowing hard, and in the distance I could hear wind chimes clanging excitedly.

Approaching the door, I hesitated and then knocked quickly. Brianna opened the door with a certain shyness. Brianna asked to follow her in the living room, while she went to look for a bottle of mineral water. She sat opposite to me, her first question was something she probably had prepared the whole night for me "I read so much about the G-spot, will its stimulation help with my relationship with men?"

"G-spot" is easier to say than Dr. Ernst Gräfenberg's last name. He was the German gynecologist who discovered the G-spot in the 1940s while researching birth control. Gräfenberg noted that the G-spot is bean shaped and basically a second clitoris. In the 1960s, Masters and Johnson reported that only clitoral stimulation and thrusting caused orgasms in women, but in 1982, the book *The G Spot and Other Discoveries about Human Sexuality,* by Americans Alice Khan Ladas, Beverly Whipple, and John D. Perry, came out. This was the first book that defined the location of the G-spot, as well as proved its existence. In 2008, Italian researchers used ultrasound to prove that G-spot orgasms were vaginal.

How To Find Her G-spot

The G-spot is not actually a spot but an area approximately 1 inch in diameter known scientifically as the Skene's glands. The G-spot is located about 1½ to 3 inches inside the vagina and is described as being behind the pubic bone. It appears that every woman has one, although some are more difficult to locate than others.

You will find that the G-spot is slightly rough, ridged like the top of your mouth, and contains a very large bundle of nerves. Medically, this is referred to as the urethral sponge; this tissue is similar to that of a penis (*see drawing: Scientists increasingly call the Skene's glands the "female prostate" because they make secretions that are almost identical to the seminal fluid produced by the male prostate in chapter 7*) and may feel like a small bean under your finger. It usually can be felt on the upper wall of the vagina (when a woman is lying on her back) halfway to the cervix and feels like a small hump on the pubic bone that swells as it is stimulated. In fact, the G-spot swells only under stimulation, and this is why for years so many doctors never felt it.

When the G-spot is first stimulated, you may feel as if you need to urinate, even if you have emptied your bladder in advance. Use the fingers of one hand to touch the anterior wall or roof of the vagina, and press the other hand against your mons pubis. After some time, the urge to urinate will disappear, and a very pleasurable sensation will take its place. After a while, the G-spot will swell and erect, filling the whole vaginal cavity. (*see drawing: After a while, the G-spot will swell and erect, filling the whole vaginal cavity*)

The G-spot swell because of the Skene's glands. The Skene's glands, sometime called the lesser vestibular periurethral (or paraurethral) glands, are located on the upper wall of the vagina around the lower end of the urethra. They drain into the urethra near the urethral opening by some openings called ducts. The tissues that surround these glands include part of the clitoris, which, as you will remember, swells with blood and reaches up inside the vagina under sexual stimulation or arousal.

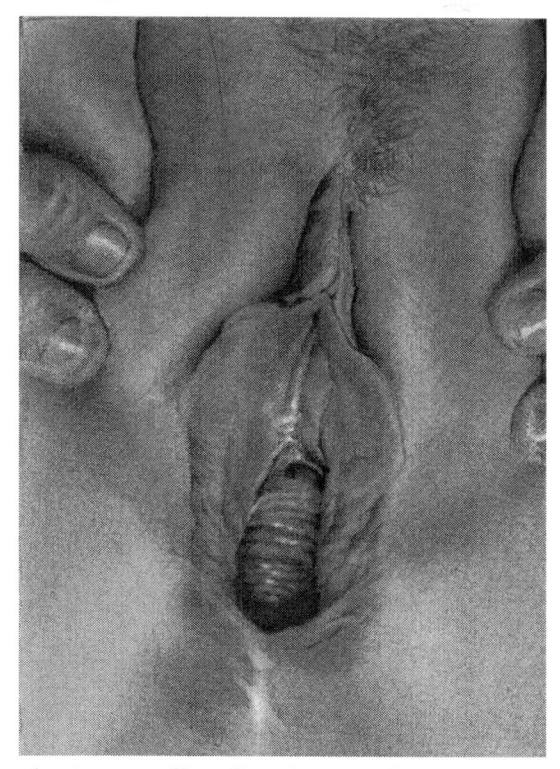

After a while, the G-spot will swell and erect, filling the whole vaginal cavity

Scientists increasingly call the Skene's glands the "female prostate" because they make secretions that are almost identical to the seminal fluid produced by the male prostate. (*see drawing: Scientists increasingly call the Skene's glands the "female prostate" because they make secretions that are almost identical to the seminal fluid produced by the male prostate*)

Stimulation of the G-spot, an area about as large as a quarter, increases the size of the Skene's glands' spongy tissue situated to the left and right of the urethral orifice. Under stimulation, the Skene's glands swell with blood just as a penis does. The Skene's glands' thirty-two ducts open into the urethral canal. At the beginning, female ejaculation may be small in volume and may increase with the time, also becoming more and more enjoyable for the woman. The glands seem to behave much like a household sponge, which, as it swells and becomes bigger, has the possibility of handling more and more fluid, which also squirts out more easily with use.

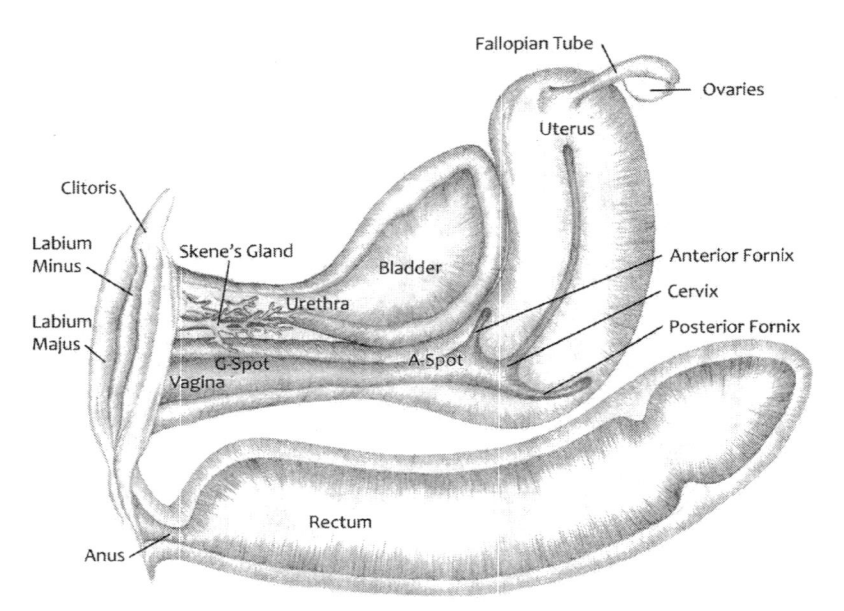

Scientists increasingssly call the Skene's glands the "female prostate" because they make secretions that are almost identical to the seminal fluid produced by the male prostate

Steps for Finding the G-Spot

1. An empty bladder is advisable.

2. Position your partner on her back with knees bent toward her face and parted.

3. Feet should be flat.

4. A pillow under her buttocks will make her more comfortable.

5. Arousal makes the G-spot easier to find; thus use a lot of foreplay.
6. Use a lot of lubrication.
7. Go as slowly as possible.
8. Never rush.
9. Make her very relaxed.
10. Ask her to breathe deeply.
11. Make sure your fingernails are short and very smooth.
12. Use the tip of your index finger and/or your middle finger.
13. As you cannot see the G-spot, use the sensitivity of the tips of your fingers to locate it.

G-Spot Response

Email received: *Dear Jean-Claude, I have had a Tantra massage before and it was a good experience; however, I was not able to have an ejaculation, I sometimes wonder if I can have one? What do you think is preventing me from having one? The main reason why I would like to have the Tantra massage, is because I have been discovering little by little my sensuality, exploring myself and learned the great power of Tantra. I am Hispanic and was married for 20 years and I do not think I ever had a good orgasm during that time....sad but it is true. Based on my culture, ignorance if you wish, kids, love, whatever..... I was not that aware of the importance of sex in my life and specially my own satisfaction. Sara .C*

Stimulation of the G-spot produces an orgasm different from that of the clitoris, it produce the ejaculation or squirting. Women usually use the word *liberation* to describe this G-spot pleasure. Some women like to find and stimulate the G-spot themselves (see Chapter 6), and others prefer to have a lover do this if they do not know where the G-spot is themselves.

All women have erogenous zones that are more sensitive than those of other women, and I certainly find that this is true of the G-spot. The G-spot, however, is also a trainable erogenous zone. This means that the more the G-spot is stimulated, the more sensitive it becomes; eventually, it will swell, but finding it for the first time may not bring forth the amount of excitement that might have been anticipated.

A man should plan on a tremendous amount of foreplay before even considering trying to find the G-spot of his partner. You should impart to her that this night is going to be very special. Take the time to massage her for 1 or 2 hours. Wait until she begs for it, and then slowly enter with your finger and explore the G-spot.

Function of the G-spot

The G-spot's function may not be solely to produce great orgasmic pleasure. We do not yet know everything about the G-spot, since its existence has been ignored for so long. I have encountered many women who could not come to orgasm unless they had several G-spot massages. These women found that they experienced female ejaculation (more about this in Chapter 10), which itself triggered a clitoral orgasm. Undoubtedly this is due to the roots of the clitoris ending in the Skene's glands.

Some women also report that during childbirth the G-spot also served a certain function. When their PC muscles were pushed out during the final phase of childbirth, several women told me, they experienced pleasure similar to an orgasm. In addition, the G-spot has a psychological function, discussed in Chapter 8 in the section titled "The Life of a Woman Who Ejaculates."

The G-spot has been talked about since Greek antiquity. It appears always to have been controversial for men but never for the women who actually experienced the pleasures of the G-spot. This makes me wonder whether some men experience a certain jealousy, wishing to retain ejaculation for themselves.

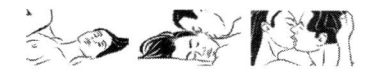

G-spot Exercise

You should know that you can indeed find the G-spot in yourself, and massage it. Knowing where it is will help you to relax when it is touched, so it's important that you not only locate it, but also, if possible, pleasure yourself with the G-spot.

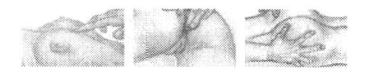

Motivational Moment

As a man, finding a woman's G-spot will make you a great lover, and your partner will truly appreciate that you took her to that new level of sexuality. Thus I encourage any man to find the G-spot in his partner.

As a woman, you will undoubtedly love this new erogenous zone. It will indeed be a new experience and the beginning of a great sensual adventure.

G-spot Self-Stimulation and Kegel Exercises

It was late October when I received the email: "I read your reviews on your website, and your massage is exactly what I need today. Do you do outcall massages? – Krystal"

This was quite a fantastic response as far as I was concerned. My website includes information about the services that I offer, along with reviews from past guests. I was pleased that Krystal had taken the time to review them.

"If you wish to be in a state of multiple orgasms for a few hours, I can do this for you," I replied. "If you want to experience female ejaculation or A- spot orgasm, then you wish to touch the core and the inner sexuality of your soul. The whole experience will be extremely spiritual, an experience you will remember forever. Allow me to massage your back and your feet, and then you will understand the power of my hands on your soul and body."

For some reason, I loved the name Krystal. It was unique and very pleasant to read. It made me think of purity and cleanliness.

"I have a business dinner tonight," came her reply, "I would like to receive your massage before that dinner. Would you be able to visit me at Marina del Rey at my private apartment? It is a large suite at the The Ritz-Carlton Hotel."

When I read this message, my heart skipped a beat. I love this little hotel along the marina overlooking the water, where I can sit for hours and watch as the boats on the water traveled endlessly. The Ritz-Carlton is also amazing from an architectural standpoint, since it is one of the older hotels in the area.

"You are looking at a two-hour-long process," I responded. "I am sure your companions will enjoy your company and your big smile. For sure they will know! Your request for a Tantric massage—is it needed for stress

relief related to some sexual frustration? Is it related to a spiritual blockage? Or do you need to achieve multiple orgasms?"

"I need multiple orgasms," Krystal replied. "I've only had two or three in my life. I'm thirty-three. I have no problems with having a single orgasm, although sometimes it takes a little while."

I explained that if she had had multiple orgasms only a few times in her life, it was because she was extremely relaxed and in love when it happened. This is often the secret of multiple orgasms. I advised Krystal to do some Kegel exercises all day, and she was fine. She did very well, actually.

Kegels for Orgasmic Pleasure

It may not be obvious, but prior to G-spot stimulation, it is advisable for you to perform Kegel exercises. These exercises, created by Dr. Arnold Kegel, allow you to work out your vaginal muscles. This will enable you to squeeze your partner's lingam and prepare you for G-spot stimulation during intercourse. Kegels are recommended because the muscles used for G-spot orgasms are your pubococcygeus (PC) muscles. These are the same muscles that you use to control the flow of urine.

Kegel exercises are the most important for female sexuality. Strong PC muscles will bring you an enhanced sex life, better childbirth, enhanced sexual energy, and, in your middle and old age, much better control of your urine. Kegel exercises will help a woman to become a fantastic lover and are a first step in becoming multi orgasmic.

A number of different aids are available for Kegel exercises:

- Miniature barbells.
- Balls of different types. Metal balls are better because they are heavier, and you can use them all day long very discreetly. *(see picture in Chapter 4: Metal balls)*

- Scissor-type aids such as the Kegelmaster (*see picture in Chapter 4: The Kegelmaster*) or Kegelexerciser.

Working the Correct Muscles

If you insert fingers into your vagina and concentrate on squeezing them, you should be able to feel which muscles you used. If you are unsure, concentrate on the muscles you use to stop the flow of urine the next time you urinate. Both males and females naturally squeeze these muscles for bladder and bowel control.

Contract these muscles for 5 seconds, and then relax for 5, eventually building up to 10 seconds. Strengthening any muscle works best when exercise is repetitive, so the exercises should be repeated 100 to 200 times per day. Some women do them while watching TV, driving, or simply relaxing.

While you are doing your Kegel exercises, start to breathe slowly, and release slowly. Focusing your mind on something very positive such as the best part of the universe (perhaps under a crystalline waterfall) or visualizing a love fountain running out of your urethra can help. Within a few weeks of starting Kegels, women often report to me that they can have an orgasm just by pushing their PC muscles up and down.

Preparing for Self-Stimulation

Since G-spot stimulation feels better and the spot itself is easier to locate if you are aroused, you might try watching a stimulating movie online or read a few passages of your favorite erotic book. Simply using imagination as well as fantasies can sexually excite some women, bringing them a rush of sexual energy. Arousal helps the female prostate to build up its supply of liquid, brought forth by the engorgement (swelling) of surrounding tissues with blood.

Positions

1. A majority of women will lie on their backs, with their knees slightly bent and their legs somewhat widely separated.

2. Having pillows behind your head so that you do not need to raise your upper body to reach deeply inside is helpful. Another pillow under your buttocks is also recommended.

3. You may find that it's easier to reach deep within yourself if you lie on your non dominant side, taking the fetal position with your knees tight against your chest.

4. Other women tell me that it's best if they squat, perhaps in the bathtub, to perform self G-spot stimulation; after all, ejaculation, when it occurs, is 3 percent urine, so it's best to keep it off of carpets, chairs, and sofas.

5. Even if you create a lot of your own lubrication, you may find it more exciting to use additional lubricant. Be sure to choose a water-based lube to avoid any possible allergic reaction.

6. You should avoid

    - Glycerin-based lubes (possibility of yeast infections).

    - Oil-based lubes (destroys latex condoms).

    - Silicone-based lubes (destroys other silicones and some women may be allergic to them).

Movement and Pressure

1. Push either one or two fingers into your vagina aligned with its front side.

2. Apply a bit of pressure, because the G-spot is actually deep in your vaginal wall.

3. Finger movement can be side to side or top to bottom, once you find the ridged surface.

4. You may use a mirror to locate your G-spot if you wish.

5. With one hand, separate the lips of your vagina widely, and after you are aroused push hard with your pelvic and PC muscles.

6. If you observe that the upper portion of your vagina has a variegated appearance, you have actually seen your G-spot!

Toys for G-spot Stimulation

There are a great number of toys available—the majority of which are curved vibrators—for reaching your G-spot properly. Be sure and aim the curve toward your belly button, use some lube, and ensure you are already aroused when you utilize these toys. Arousal plus some lube will aid an easy insertion.

Single women find that using toys enables them to have G-spot orgasms. Combined with clitoral orgasms, these will also be awakening orgasms that will liberate your sexual energy.

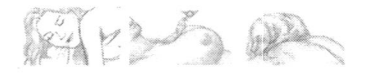

Motivational Moment

Tantric teaching frees up your sexuality. It offers you a means of surrendering to the moment, of becoming empowered, centered, and very relaxed. Through Tantra, you will learn to release fears and other emotions, be present, breathe, and totally relax. Your whole life will start to change: You will start to feel happier, and your skin will be clearer. This is due to the phenomenon of female ejaculation, the release of the fluid that gives you such cosmic pleasure. You will feel like you are making love with the universe.

Pleasure produced by the G-spot are more of a whole-body experience than the intense burst of pleasure experienced with a clitoral orgasm. Your pleasure will begin deep inside, and then it will rise throughout your entire body. The contractions are actually stronger and seem to last much longer than those of a clitoral orgasm. The great advantage is that this pleasure will last as long as your G-spot is stimulated.

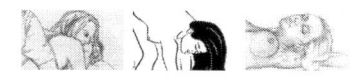

Note About the A-spot, G-Spot and Kegels

In this chapter you gained knowledge of a largely unknown, sensitive spot called the A-spot. Stimulation of the A-spot, as well as being the key to opening the door for multiple orgasms, has the power to give ecstatic pleasure. When stimulated, the A-spot's highly sensitive tissue, located at the inside end of the vaginal tube between the cervix and bladder, will generate fierce orgasmic contractions that then lead to delirious pleasure.

This chapter also emphasized the G-spot as a new erogenous zone, explaining its history and function, along with how to find it. Now that you have learned about the G-spot, it is imperative that you keep looking, ladies, for you'll agree that it's supremely important to eventually reach different types of pleasure!

Strong PC muscles, you learned, are very important in stimulation of the G-spot and to the additional pleasure available in this way. You learned how to exercise these muscles with Kegels, and you've also learned a number of positions that can be utilized for G-spot self-stimulation. In the next chapter, you will discover the psychological importance for women of female ejaculation. Women of all sexual orientations, with or without a partner, will be able to use this information to continue on their way to the nadir of orgasmic pleasure. Keep it up!

Fill in this log to record the results of your exercises:

1. Which of the A-spot, G-spot, and Kegel exercises did you do this week?

2. What change do you want to see in yourself, spiritually and sexually?

3. How do you feel about your own sexuality, now that you have done these exercises?

4. On a scale of 1 to 10, with 10 the maximum, how have these exercises improved the quality of your orgasm(s)?

	1	2	3	4
Week 1				
Week 2				
Week 3				
Week 4				
Week 5				
Week 6				
Week 7				
Week 8				

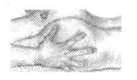

CHAPTER 8

The Fountain of Love: Female Ejaculation

Observation and my own life experience tell me that we often simply accept the way life goes. There is certainly more for us than just accepting. This is the reason why so many women have sexual tension and problems. They simply accept that a man will only do what pleases him. If they expected and demanded a little more, their sexual satisfaction as well as his could be met.

Before me the pane on the window began to fog. I turned away and returned to my trusty desk. This was the place where I allowed women into my world and started to help them with their problems.

I had a voice mail. The voice was sweet and low. Almost always, women leave their messages using a very sexy voice. I caught the last part of the message: "I have become detached from my womanly body through the stress of modern life. I feel blocked energetically and disconnected from my true sexual self. When I read your advert, it seemed like the perfect solution. I have never had a Tantric massage before and am curious as to what happens."

"However, I have experienced female ejaculation a few times," her voice went on, "and I can make myself ejaculate sometimes through masturbation with my G-spot vibrator. If it is important to you, I have blue-green

eyes, plus a beautiful smile. I'm young and have a great body. Have done lots of acting for television and the big screen. I am a very positive person, a happy human and feel you may bring a very positive experience in my sexual life. Please come any time today. I will wait for you."

Then she left her address and phone number, and her name: "Grace."

On my way to Grace's place, I thought out loud about how modern life makes us into robots. Survival is such a problem that we have lost pleasure and spirituality. Tantra sees our physical pleasure as deeply connected to our spirituality. The center of our pleasure is in our brains, and the brain is also connected to the cosmos. When we release positive thoughts throughout the universe through sexual pleasure, it makes our planet a better place.

Grace opened the door eagerly, smiling shyly at me. Those blue-green eyes gazed into mine. She led me silently into her house. Words would spoil the sensuality of the moment, but she had made sure the house had a nice atmosphere for us. The curtains were drawn against the wicked storm, and several scented candles were placed strategically around the room. The soft aroma of lavender drifted over my body, tickling my nostrils with its flowery scent.

There was one thing that can be said about Grace: She certainly was open to the experience and willing to offer herself to whatever came from it. I had been surprised by how quickly she had provided me with her information.

Without notice, Grace undid the bow that tied her white cotton sundress together, and I easily slipped the dress up and over her head, leaving her in just a tiny pair of underwear. She whispered into my ear, "I want you to make me soak my bed."

Love's energy is one that grows within, and with Tantric lovemaking, the physical movements, our breathing, the sounds we make, and the presence of that energy are all the means of expanding that very specific ecstatic energy so that it can extend to the rest of the body. Lovemaking does not release energy; it just takes ecstasy and bliss and expands it. Female sexual energy is boundless, considering women's ability to host life and experience what seems to be limitless bliss.

Female ejaculation has throughout history picked up a plethora of names. For instance, Tantra calls it "Amrita." Those who are poetically or romantically inclined call it the "Fountain of Love," classical mythology refers to it either as the "Greek Nectar of Aphrodite" or as the "Fountain of Venus," and the French call it the "Champagne of Sex." Today, women refer to it as "splashing," "spraying," "spurting," or "squirting," but in the end, no matter what it is called, it is still female ejaculation.

Female ejaculation is a great pleasure; it is an important step in the woman sexuality. However, so many women told me, female ejaculation is great, I love it but I do not feel like an orgasm. Other told me it cannot be compared, it is not like the bang of an orgasm it is felt more like pleasure from all over the body. A vaginal orgasm occurs when there is a strong contraction of the PC muscles affecting the clitoris's roots in the Skene's glands. Some women may have a vaginal orgasm without a female ejaculation. Today, we know that the fluid of the female ejaculation is from the wall of the bladder but not from the bladder cavity itself. Then that fluid is stored for a moment in the Skene's gland then pushed out of the urethral opening. Some women have always ejaculated easily, and they find that the art of foreplay—touching, nibbling, massaging, stroking, and licking—was created to activate the female body and ready it for ejaculation. Perhaps these lucky women may have been embarrassed to ejaculate in the beginning, yet most probably quickly understood that this was the right way to be. On the other hand, some women may ejaculate strictly "by accident," because they are intensely relaxed. Perhaps they were with their boyfriends in a very romantic setting, or maybe they were masturbating, and it just happened. Still others will need to learn all about how to make female ejaculation happen. The more free you are with your mind, at easy with your body and open to your sexuality, the more easily female ejaculation will happen. For my readers who want to learn more about female ejaculation, please read my book: The Confessions of a Hollywood Tantra Masseur.

Stimulation from a Partner

For several reasons, female ejaculation has been pushed aside in our modern world. Some women sex therapists have avoided or criticized the subject because they themselves never have experienced that kind of pleasure. Some doctors still believe that female ejaculation is a medical condition. As a man, I can see that in our macho world, some men may feel that the word *ejaculation* has been hijacked from them by those who advocate female supremacy. Also, it can takes so much trust and time to reach a state of readiness for female ejaculation that with today's world rushing by, most lovers can no longer spend the time needed with their partners that would allow the woman to reach this crescendo of pleasure. This also may apply to a vagina orgasm or even clitoral orgasm, since many men suffer of premature ejaculation, they don't have much time to give pleasure to their partner, since they are so preoccupied by their own orgasm.

Achieving this degree of sexual energy takes time, so it is exceedingly important not to rush and allow it to develop correctly. With some women, this may mean using two fingers to massage the G-spot carefully; others may be involved with a man whose lingam or penis is large, long or curved so that it naturally rubs against that spot, or

Sex: Woman First

they may have accidentally discovered that a certain position will give them the needed contact.

No matter how female ejaculation is accomplished, both the woman and the man need to understand that it will sometimes take time; it may take between a few days to a few weeks. If a woman doesn't ejaculate, it is because she is not ready, so do not push her. If you massage her for 5 to 10 minutes each time you have intercourse, female ejaculation *will* happen. You may stimulate her slowly with the tips of your fingers, making circles or a figure 8, and then change to a more vigorous and stronger "come here" motion with your fingers. (*see drawing: You may stimulate her slowly with the tips of your fingers, making circles or a figure 8, and then change to a more vigorous and stronger "come here" motion with your fingers*) Because the Skene's glands need to be stimulated, if your woman is multiple orgasmic, bringing her to orgasm first will make female ejaculation easier. If she is not orgasmic at all, female ejaculation could cause her to have an orgasm from the clitoral zone.

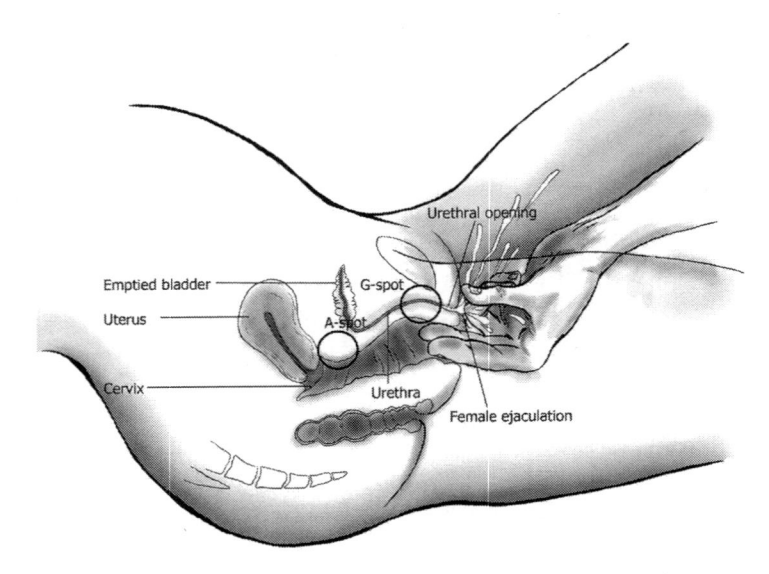

You may stimulate her slowly with the tips of your fingers, making circles or a figure 8, and then change to a more vigorous and stronger "come here" motion with your fingers

Everything has to be right: In the beginning, the woman will need to push with her PC muscles, breathe correctly, and totally relax. But very quickly all of this will begin to happen naturally in a very synchronized way. Then she needs to let go and get beyond the feeling that she may urinate, simply enjoying the feelings that will come. Once she ejaculates the first time, it is easier for her to ejaculate once again. When the stimulation happens again, her mind and muscles know what to do to get that pleasure. It becomes a reflex. With time as well as practice, that spongy erectile tissue will erect whenever she is aroused and stimulated. The G-spot area will swell and may fill the entire vaginal entrance, so that her partner need only caress that erect tissue gently for her to begin to ejaculate once more.

For some women, it is best to stimulate the A-spot at the same time as the G-spot, while others would rather have the clitoris orally stimulated while the G-spot is stimulated with the fingers. Still others like oral stimulation of the clitoris at the same time that a vibrator is used to stimulate the G-spot. The point is, there are various combinations and possibilities, and each depends upon the individual woman.

You will find that female ejaculation does not always require direct manual stimulation of the G-spot. Indeed, some of the paraurethral or Skene's glands react well to oral stimulation or even to a state of mental arousal, responding with ejaculation. The fact that some women can ejaculate without even being touched once more proves that the brain is the most important sex organ!

Some of the most wonderful feelings will come from having the A-spot stimulated along with the G-spot and U-spot, and even the clitoris—either alternately or simultaneously (*see drawing: You may stimulate her slowly with the tips of your fingers, making circles or a figure 8, and then change to a more vigorous and stronger "come here" motion with your fingers*).

By combining stimulation of three or four of the magic spots at the same time, you will be able to produce fierce orgasmic contractions that may lead to delirious pleasure and female ejaculation.

A few months after your Goddess will have started to ejaculate, you will notice that her G-spot gets swollen very easily as soon as she get aroused. You won't need to go deep to look for her G-spot. Her G-spot will now take up the whole space at the opening of the vagina. You will just have to caress that swollen G-spot gently with the tip of your finger to make her ejaculate.

Email to Jean-Claude

- The first time I was a little obsessed with learning how to do it and then I met a guy who claimed he was an expert at it. Because it takes me so long to orgasm, I put him to the test. Within 5 minutes I squirted. It didn't feel like an orgasm though. He was able to do it over and over and he kind of taught me how to do it, and I've been able to make the girl squirt ever since. My boyfriend now also knew how to do it. It takes more than 5 minutes with him, but he does it and it feels more like an orgasm than it did with the other guy. I usually stop it right as its about to happen, but when I let it go - there is a decent amount. Yvonne P.

Freeway to G-spot Massage

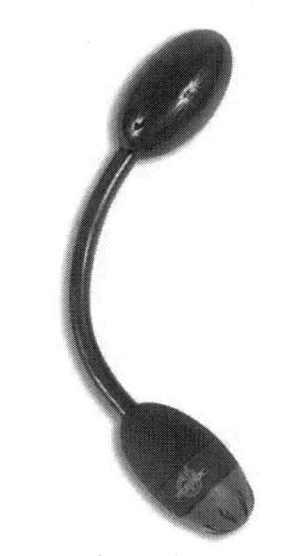

Flex-a-pleasure

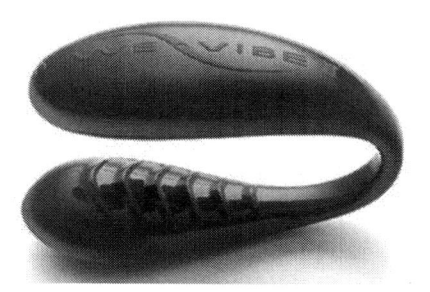

Wev2 We Vibe 2

A less romantic approach (for the lover who wants to take a short cut in order to be sure of pleasuring) to stimulate the G-spot would be to use two vibrators. For this, choose a G-spot vibrator with a flexible vibrating handle such as the Flex-a-pleasure or the Wev2 We Vibe 2 (*see picture of the vibrator Flex-a-pleasure, Wev2 We Vibe 2*) and a high-speed vibrator such as the Hitachi Wand Massager (*see picture of the vibrator Hitachi Wand Massager*) for the clitoris or a nearby spot. This technique often will bring a woman to female ejaculation or at least a very strong orgasm from the clitoris area. If you apply this technique, I promise she will ask you to do it again and again. You can become her God , with simply two vibrators.

Every individual is different, of course, and just as men do not make love the same way to every woman, every woman does not react in the same way with each man she encounters sexually. The act of lovemaking also involves chemistry and emotion; and as her partner, it is up to you to determine the best way to stimulate your woman's G-spot and give her the most pleasurable result possible. Each step is a beautiful journey. In traveling it, you will learn a tremendous amount about your partner, as well as about yourself.

The intensity of female ejaculation is entirely different than that of a clitoral orgasm. Female ejaculation is not better (because we all know that sexual pleasure is always beautiful!), it is just different and can best be described as being "all over." Both body and brain are involved, and so female ejaculation most accurately can be described as both a physical as well as a spiritual experience. This leaves a woman with a sense of liberation, of feeling freer, like a burden has been removed.

Female ejaculation can come and go. I have met women who experienced female ejaculation for months, only to have it disappear and then come back later on. The reason may have something to do with a woman's hormonal levels, but we also know that it may depend upon the woman's level of relaxation as well as her trust in her partner or emotional state at the time. I regularly receive emails from women who say, "*I used to have female ejaculation but have not been able to recreate that pleasure. I am longing for a lover to make me feel that way again.*"

For a long time, women have been preoccupied with whether the fluid that they ejaculate is urine or not, and often a woman may think that there is no way she's going to pee in the bed in front of her partner. If this sounds like the case for you, my recommendation is that the man should tell the woman that she will feel adorably sexy when she does so, and that it is just fine if she pees in front of you. You will have to tell her to simply let go and be herself.

Female ejaculate may contain as much as 3 percent urine— sometimes more—but it is never urine alone. Although it may change in texture and color as well as odor, generally the ejaculate is clear and tastes like water. For her first time, the quantity will be only a dribble, but with time she will instinctively learn to push her PC muscles, and the ejaculate will become more and more copious, bringing with it additional pleasure. The amount of ejaculate may vary from a few drops to 2 or 3 cups. (Should you desire a strong ejaculation, you should be prepared to work your PC muscles one hundred times, three times per day, as described in Chapter 7).

During the first three or four months of experiencing female ejaculation, some women have asked me, "*That's it? This is not a big deal!*". Then, gradually, they learn to like it, and slowly they learn that pleasure empowers the body. Of course, other women tell me from the first day that ejaculation is just great, and I hear comments such as, "*I feel as if I've had a total liberation of my body!*".

I honestly cannot say that a female ejaculation is better than a clitoral climax. As a man, I have no idea! I do listen to women, however, and although their comments make me think that female ejaculation is different and special, all types of orgasms are clearly very pleasurable. Some women do say, "*I tried it, but it's not for me*", and this too is just fine.

Times When the G-spot is Extra Sensitive

A number of variations occur in the female human body, such as fluctuating estrogen levels, which may affect the G-spot. The G-spot will be less sensitive, for instance, when you have more estrogen in your body. For example, if a female is older than thirty, she may have greater G-spot sensitivity because she will normally expect to have lower estrogen levels. In this circumstance, the vaginal wall will be thinner, and the spot will be easier to manipulate.

For the same reason, your G-spot may be more sensitive just prior to your menstrual cycle. Let's look at it this way: A few days before a woman's normal period, her feminine body is readying for conception. Her body experiences a heightened sex drive at this time, making her more sensitive during coitus. Since the body is already quite turned on at such times, the G-spot probably is already sensitized.

Trust Needed

When I look at the result of the quiz I send to my clients at http://mysecretquiz.com/index.php

- 17% I have only one orgasm when I masturbate or through intercourse.
- 33% I don't have an orgasm with my partner.
- 51% I never have an orgasm from vaginal penetration
- 58% No, I have not experienced female ejaculation

Why do women not achieve female ejaculation or even a simple orgasm? Most women are self conscious of their body, and many women wrote to me saying "*I am a giver., I am bored when my partner try to give oral, I would rather be giving to him and most of the time I stop him."* The problem is, most women think about everything they have done during the day and all the chores waiting for them tomorrow: do the laundry, teacher meeting, meeting with her boss. And also, a woman thinks too much about performing. She thinks so much about her orgasm, and worries if she is going to be able to achieve one or not. She is so focused that often, the orgasm start and before it reaches the peak, the energy break and go down, and it is over. The solution for you, the man: you need to give her a lot of foreplay to relax her mind, then she will feel that you know what you are doing and she will trust you and open completely.

Reaching female ejaculation requires a tremendous amount of trust in a partner because the woman will feel extremely vulnerable. To reach the level of ejaculation, she needs to clear her mind and surrender control of her sexuality. She is now totally in your hands and will feel naked—and not just in a physical sense—in front of you. Only if she feels perfectly safe will her level of trust be high enough that she can totally let go.

Remember, it is a great sign of trust if she can relax that much with you. Do not abuse that trust, but make sure that you show your appreciation for what she did for you. Take her surrender as what it is: a great present. Additionally, as a man, do not make female ejaculation *your* goal. If it does happen, do not crow about it, but instead consider it as something precious between the two of you.

Psychological Effect of Female Ejaculation

Physically, a female orgasm with ejaculation will release endorphins, which psychologically relaxes the portions of the brain that dwell on anxiety and fear. It also causes the release of serotonin, which brings with it a calming effect. In addition, a female ejaculation produces a high level of immunoglobulin-A, which makes her feel good and fights off infections.

Sexual Healing

The first time that a woman experiences female ejaculation, she may feel very fragile, and any past traumas of her life, especially sexual ones, may come to the forefront. She may feel that a deep secret has been divulged.

Shame, guilt, pain, betrayals, hurts, and past traumas related to sexuality all can obstruct the way to a woman's sexual fulfillment, orgasmic potential, bliss, and ecstasy. Although science knows better, today's society teaches us to suppress emotions. Suppression, however, builds up "emotional blocks" in our bodies over time, and this causes energy blocks. These are the same reasons that the chakras can be closed.

These energy blocks, when related to a woman's sexual feelings, are specifically held in the area of the G-spot. Unfortunately, these blocks may obstruct her ability to experience sexual pleasure, orgasms, and multiple orgasms. The more a woman ejaculates, the more she cleans up the blockage-creating traumas. A woman who was raped as a teenager told me, "*Ejaculating saved me ten years of going to the shrink.*"

A woman may have sexual wounds and issues that cause her to simply go numb or basically shut down during sex. With the use of the Tantric connection to the higher energy of sex, female ejaculation may turn into a healing and cleansing process. Ejaculating is not only erotic but also very cleansing. You will feel it as a deep surrender, and you will become very in tune with yourself and others and exceedingly centered. This happens especially at the beginning, before ejaculation occurs the first time. One woman told me, "*It was as if I saw my whole sex life in front of me like a movie. I had flashbacks of some of my sexual activities—bad memories and good memories. I felt as though I were coming home, or becoming a woman, until everything cleared up and I began to ejaculate."*

The Life of the Woman Who Ejaculates

To be known as a great lover, whether you are a man or a woman, is very personal between partners and is a question of chemistry as well as of emotion. A woman does not have to have a female ejaculation to be a great lover. A woman may explore ejaculation out of curiosity about what her body may be able to offer her in the matter of her pleasure. I have encountered women who could experience female ejaculation but not clitoral orgasms. Eventually, from receiving the pleasure of female ejaculation, the ability to have a clitoral orgasm grew.

I have met a woman who had separated from her husband, but because he read about female ejaculation online and they changed their lovemaking and relationship, today they are perfectly happy together. I also met a woman who divorced because she met a lover who made her feel the pleasures of the G-spot and another whose husband divorced her because he disliked the fact that she ejaculated in bed and had to sleep on a soaked mattress. Everyone has a different tale to tell.

Do not work at female ejaculation in order to please your lover or because you feel it looks sexy. Work on it because you wish to share something extremely intimate with your partner. Do it because you wish to give something back in union with him to the universe, and because you wish to reach a new level of consciousness with sex. You see, this is a high level of Tantra, if you know how to utilize it. It is truly magic sex!

A woman who ejaculates regularly will become more and more positive and secure about her sexuality. She will have a beautiful smile upon her face and will attract love all around her because she projects love and positive energy. She will feel that everything around her is great. Unfortunately, if she stops ejaculating, either because she doesn't have a partner or her present partner do not know how to stimulate her, or she lose interest about her own sexuality, then she will return to the same lethargy of earlier times, with all the normal worries that we have in our daily lives. Sometimes, she may not even remember how she used to feel sexually. A woman who called me for a G-spot massage told me, *"I did not remember what I was missing."* This is like land missing water becomes a dry area. But as soon the irrigation system starts functioning again, the flowers will blossom again. Female ejaculation is "the magic key" for couples who have the right level of spiritual, emotional and sexual energy and are looking for an indestructible bond. It is a beautiful secret that no woman want to share with anyone accept her lover.

The Fountain of Love Exercise

If you do not have a partner, please go back to the last chapter and the section on Self G-spot Stimulation. If you have a partner, then it is time to share this chapter. In fact, it is time to say to him or her, *"Please, tonight I want to feel you explore me deeper! I am all yours."*

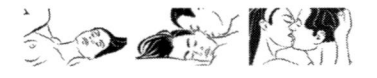

Motivational Moment

Expanding your erotic potential has been your dream. Your journey has been both precious and exhilarating, and with practice you will own it! Experiencing the Fountain of Love is an opportunity to expand your sexual energy to another level. Once it has been experienced, most women say, "*I knew there was something else inside of me, but I did not know how to find it. I am glad that your advice helped me to experience that beautiful pleasure that is now utilizing my whole body as well as my brain!*"

More than physical pleasure, female ejaculation creates a wonderful bond of love with the person who makes you feel that way for the first time.

Note About the Fountain of Love

In this chapter, you learned some of the more descriptive words that have been used for female ejaculation and how great it made other women feel when they experienced it. You have learned what female ejaculate comprises and why G-spot sensitivity varies in your own body, which has inspired you to find out more. By arriving at this chapter, you already have accomplished so much. It doesn't matter if you do or do not ejaculate yet. What matters is that you are more and more aware of what your body has to offer to pleasure you.

Fill in this log to record of the results of your exercises:

1. Which of these exercises did you do this week: exploration of your A-Spot, self G-spot stimulation, the freeway to G-spot massage with two vibrators, or something else?

2. What change do you want to see in yourself spiritually and sexually?

3. How do you feel about your own sexuality now that you have done these exercises?

4. On a scale of 1 to 10, with 10 the maximum, how have these exercises improved the quality of your orgasm(s)?

	1	2	3	4
Week 1				
Week 2				
Week 3				
Week 4				
Week 5				
Week 6				
Week 7				
Week 8				

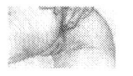

CHAPTER 9

How Women Can Become Multiple Orgasmic

The word *orgasm* refers to an intense feeling of sexual pleasure that can occur during sexual activity with a partner or during masturbation. This pleasure is experienced as a series of muscular contractions in the lower pelvic and genital area in both men and women. Women are said to be able to reach multiple orgasms, and for some it is easy to climax, or come, over and over again.

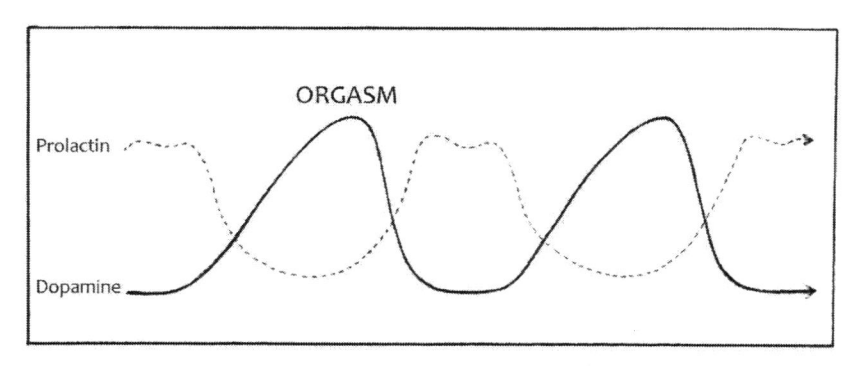

When orgasm happens, dopamine plummets, but instantly prolactin increases and counteracts dopamine.

Since the work of Masters and Johnson in 1965 and John D. Perry on the G-spot in 2006, we are still researching on the topic of multiple orgasms. Some scientists have diagnosed the inability to experience them as something to do with the position of certain nerves in the spinal cord, whereas some psychologists relate such an inability to a traumatic experience in the childhood. The latest research indicates that our pleasure and orgasm are due to a chemical call dopamine, which is behind all our needs and desires; eating, gambling, playing computer games, shopping, sexual desire. But to moderate our behavior, a second hormone is produced, called prolactin, also known as luteotropic hormone. When an orgasm happens, dopamine plummets, but instantly prolactin increases and counteracts dopamine. (*see drawing: When orgasm happens, dopamine plummets, but instantly prolactin increases and counteracts dopamine.*) This shuts off the orgasm, too give a feel sexually satisfied. We noticed that women who are using sexual orgasm to unload their stress in their marital situation have headache after intercourse or masturbation. This is due to high level of prolactin and low level of dopamine. While we are sleeping, prolactin is plummeting. Women and men who have faster sexual recovery is because they have low prolactin level, thus the prolaction doesn't go to cross the dopamine and kill the orgasm. There is a third hormone call testosterone which is also important for the arousal of the genital part of the woman as well as a correlation with a great orgasm. I would therefore suggest having your hormonal level of prolactin, dopamine and testosterone tested before feeling guilty about any emotional type of blockage or incrimination of your partner or yourself. If everything is normal then the reason for any difficulty to welcome sex could be because of need to stay in control of her sexuality.

Often women are contacting me asking if a Tantric massage would change their sex life from an absence of orgasm when they masturbate or a nonexistent libido, to a multi orgasmic level. Tantra will teach you to trust each other and become closer to each other. A woman may cut off her orgasm prematurely because she wants to stay in control. To stay in control is a second nature for a woman; she programs herself to stay in control of her sexuality. She may wish to stay in control because she doesn't wish to become vulnerable to a man with whom she is not sure of his emotion or if he is emotionally weak. If she become vulnerable, some men will use their women and abuse them. She may have seen the same thing happen to her mother. Her mother was so much in love with her father or step father, and then the bastard was abusing her. She put a little mental note in her mind that no way this will happen to me. Also, she may wish to stay in control because she doesn't want to be pregnant. She learn to stay alert and never relax during the intercourse. To stay in control is so much part of her, that at this end she never relax even with her husband or her most closest lover and doesn't remember when all this begun. For some women it may take time to trust her man, but sometime it is completely instantly. It cannot be explained, the chemistry is there. Just looking at him, feeling him or being touched by him, and a strong bond is born forever. No wonder why some women cannot orgasm with some men but find one with whom she is completely open to her sexual pleasure.

Having multi orgasms is a dream come true for many women. If you read this chapter and apply it step by step in your sexual life, your own dream may also come true. In order to understand why some women have multi orgasms while others do not, you have to first understand that women have a specific route for sexual excitation. Imagine a curve that follows these stages (*see: Imagine a curve that follows these stages*)

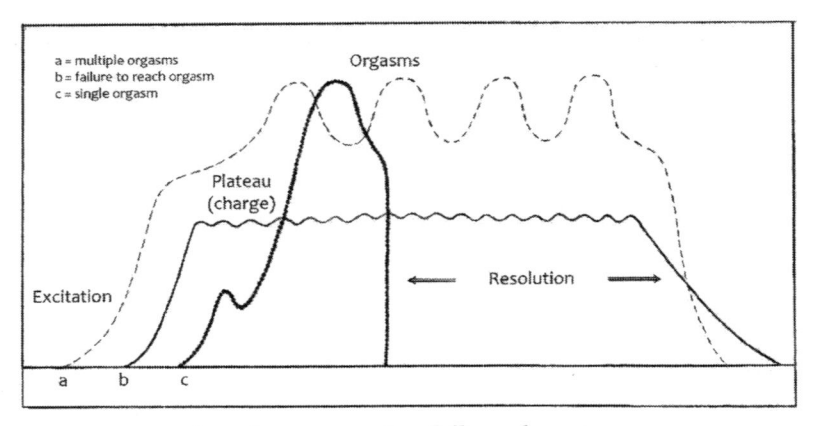

Imagine a curve that follows these stages

- Arousal
- Plateau
- Loss of control
- Point of no return
- Orgasm
- Plateau
- Relaxation

Foreplay is responsible for the first stage and is mandatory in all sexual acts with the aim of providing pleasure and sexual satisfaction for both partners.

In the plateau stage, the sexual energy gathered during arousal accumulates, and breathing accelerates. In this stage, in order to prolong your sexual act and accumulate even more energy (for a more explosive orgasm) before the climax, you can use the breathing techniques described in Chapter 2 to relax and contain your excitation. (*see drawing: In the plateau stage, the sexual energy gathered during arousal accumulates, and breathing accelerates*)

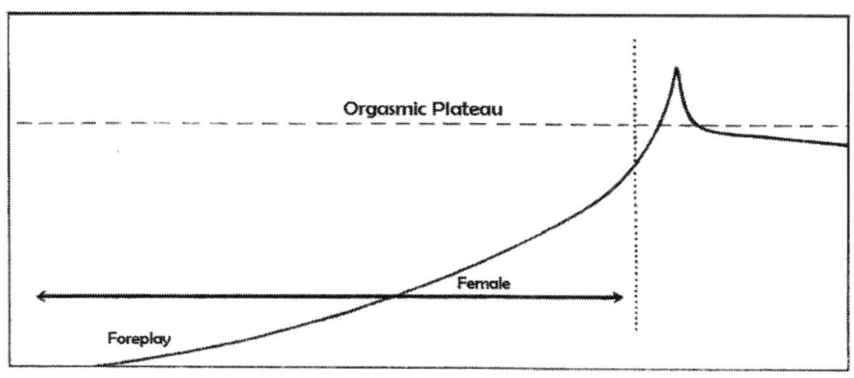

The Arousal Pattern of Women
In the plateau stage, the sexual energy gathered during arousal accumulates, and breathing accelerates

Next comes the "losing control" phase, during which, if you are relaxed and open, your body will take over, and you may start to shiver, twitch, or grab the sheets or your partner's hands or face.

Shortly after this comes the "point of no-return," that moment of maximum excitation when you feel you are about to explode. This is the perfect moment when making love, if your partner intuits this stage before you get there, for continued stimulation in order for an explosive orgasm and female ejaculation to occur.

After the "point of no return," which lasts only seconds, comes orgasm, a complete sexual, emotional, and spiritual discharge. After the orgasm, the plateau phase starts: Your clitoris and labia may begin to reduce their swelling, but you are still aroused.

If you or your partner stops stimulation, the plateau stage will last until all of your aroused spots (nipples, clitoris, anus, vagina) go back to their normal, unexcited state. The relaxation phase soon follows. If, however, you restart sexual stimulation during the plateau phase before arriving at the relaxation stage, your body will reenter the sexual curve—arousal, plateau, losing control, orgasm, plateau, and so on—as long or as many times as both of you last. This choice to re-excite after orgasm is the single difference between women who only have one orgasm per sexual act and women who have tens of them.

There are two types of multi orgasms: consecutive and progressive. Consecutive orgasms come one after the other when a woman re-enters the excitation curve and passes through all of the stages again with very little break between them. Progressive orgasms are similar, but they tend to build on one another, gradually becoming more and more intense until the woman reaches a point of immense sexual energy that is released through one mega-explosive orgasm. Progressive orgasms like this can also lead to the experience of female ejaculation. For consecutive orgasms, you may wonder when to restart the sexual stimulation after an orgasm, so that you are not too late to re-enter the curve. Here are some tips to help you and your partner recognize when the time is right:

Your breathing rhythm decreases but it is not yet regularized.

- Your body stops shivering or stretching.
- Your PC stops its spasms.
- Your nipples get softer.
- Your clitoris is slightly less sensitive.

You should get used to listening to your body carefully. It will tell you when you are ready to get back in the game. The shorter the previous orgasm, the faster you can restart sexual stimulation and enter a new sexual curve. If you are wondering what kind of sexual stimulation you should use after the first orgasm, the answer depends on what type of orgasm you had and which parts of your body are too sensitive to touch right away. If your orgasm was obtained by stimulating the clitoris by hand or by mouth, it would probably feel too sensitive to be touched, so you should focus on arousing different parts of your body, just as you did during the initial foreplay: arms, neck, lips, back, breasts, nipples, pubic area, buttocks, legs—any area that you have already declared as being erogenous and is not intolerably sensitive at this moment. Meanwhile, while you keep your excitation high with this foreplay, your clitoris will become less swollen and less sensitive. Soon you can treat it also with some tenderness and love—by gently touching it, pushing it up and down, and playing with it in whatever way arouses and pleases you.

If your orgasm was obtained through penetration and the sexual act was not very rough, your vagina will be less sensitive and you can start the stimulation (penetration) as soon as your breathing is back to normal, using breathing exercises to achieve this. You can also add clitoral stimulation at this time for the experience of a double orgasm. It is very useful in this instance for your partner to practice sexual continence. This way you can have multiple orgasms while his penis is still erect and able to penetrate you. If he ejaculates after your first orgasm and you still want to experience multiple orgasms, you can use a vibrator or your partner can perform cunnilingus or stimulate your G and A spots with his fingers or with special curved vibrators. After he regains his strength, you can continue with intercourse and vaginal orgasms.

Progressive orgasms often come one after another, without returning to foreplay and without interrupting intercourse. Some women prefer to begin by experimenting with consecutive orgasms, and then progressive orgasms come naturally while making love. Other women have progressive orgasms naturally without putting any special effort into it. Every woman has a unique personality, body, set of feelings, and experiences unique orgasms. If you have single orgasms and want to experience being multi-orgasmic, here is a set of suggestions to bring you the long-awaited multiple orgasms. Before reading these suggestions, remember that achieving great, multiple orgasms is like achievement in any other field: the more work you put in, the more reward you get out!

Baby Steps to Go from Having One Orgasm to Having Ten Orgasms

- **Liberate yourself.** Some women find it hard to experience multiple orgasms because of their mental blockages. If you were raised in a very conservative or religious family, you might have been told that sexual pleasure is a sin or that masturbation is wrong. Maybe you have been abused or punished for expressing your sexuality. Throughout the years, while fighting these prejudices, you may have allowed yourself to experience one orgasm, but having multiples on some level may have seemed like lechery to you. In this way, you may have blocked yourself from experiencing the joy of multiple orgasms. If this is the case, you could either go to a therapist who could help you find your own beliefs about sex, or read some self-help books about accepting your sexuality..

- **Self-pleasure.** Explore your body, stimulate your erogenous and non-erogenous areas, and experience different types of touches, soft or rough. Do not be afraid of trying new positions when masturbating. Just let yourself play with your body and be curious about what works and what doesn't. This way you can find out where you are sensitive before and after an orgasm, what your signs are for an orgasm, which positions give you different kinds of pleasure, and so on. There is so much to be discovered!

- **Use that extra kick**. To attain sexual pleasure, do not be afraid to use different methods. For example, try gel enhancers. These are mint-based gels that cause a warm sensation where you apply them, stimulating the area and enhancing orgasm. They are usually applied to the clitoris and the surrounding area, making it more sensitive and aroused. Choose water-based gel enhancers, since they don't harm condoms and do not leave stains on the sheets.

- **Understand your body**. You need to have a strong connection with your body in order to know when to stop and when to start again. Pay attention to your breathing, your heartbeats, your muscles contracting, and learn to know the signals your body sends as you approach an orgasm. This way, your every sensation would be emphasized, and you can observe your orgasm while completely living it; a few seconds after the orgasm, before entering the next plateau phase, you can continue stimulation, in order to achieve a new orgasm.

- **Ask for what you want**. Trust and openness are necessary in a sexual relationship. Nobody should force you to break your boundaries; it is your choice. If you want to have multiple orgasms, you need to leave your inhibitions aside and show your partner what you like and need in bed.

- **Stimulate multiple pleasure points**. If you want complex, full-body orgasms, stimulate multiple sexual points at the same time or very close in time to each other. If you have intercourse, stimulate your clitoris and your breasts at the same time if they are particularly erogenous for you. When receiving cunnilingus, ask your partner to place his finger on your perineum (the area between the vagina and the anus) and press gently. Your orgasm will feel deeper, and you will experience waves of pleasure throughout your whole body.

- **Move your energy (Chi Kung).** Whether we are talking about one's energy, kundalini, chi or prana, the point is the same: there is a life energy that connects us all and that flows through our bodies from the moment we are conceived until death. There are 49 cultures around the world that share the same essence when it comes to their chi philosophy and practice, also known as Chi Kung (Qigong). This ancient practice, Chi Kung, helps restoring the natural balance of the body, which, in return, heals itself, both physically and spiritually. You can use Chi Kung to activate your energy and move it through your body, to different areas that need more energy to be awoken. This can easily be used by women that need to connect with their bodies, to increase their sexual appetite and the intensity of their orgasms. Here is a simple exercise that you can practice to get in touch with your chi:

- To have a first contact with your chi, firmly rub your palms together, until they become warm. Then spread them apart slowly about an inch, and bring them closer again. You will feel like an air cushion between your palms. You could feel tingles or a slight pressure. That is your energy, the Chi, moving from one hand to the other.

- Use your breath and focus on your chi. When you inhale, imagine a flow of energy going from the base of the spine, up the spine to your brain, and when you exhale, let it move down the front of your body in the midline, to your abdomen and sexual organs. You will feel invigorated, and maybe even aroused. While doing this, you can slowly move your pelvis back, when you inhale, and forward, when you exhale.

Chi Kung offers many techniques to gain access to your healing life energy, and you can become healthier, more balanced, more sexual and more beautiful by practicing this dance of the energy through your body.

Kegels for Multiple Orgasms

Women often overlook the benefits of Kegel exercises, but they are exceedingly important, whether you are single, heterosexual, or lesbian. Women do not always understand the real power of these exercises. We live in times of immediate rewarding where brand-new cell phones are already obsolete after three months, so Kegel exercises may seem very archaic because it takes so long to get a result.

You'll need to perform your Kegel exercises daily, keeping in mind that no one will know that you are in the midst of doing them. (See Chapter 7 for information on how to do them correctly.) Because the G-spot grows in sensitivity the more it is stimulated and the more often you utilize it, the easier it will become for you to employ it for better orgasms. Always go gently on yourself; you are not in competition within yourself to achieve an ultimate goal.

If you follow this recommendation—whether you have never had an orgasm or already have multiple orgasms—you will be overjoyed. Squeeze those muscles a hundred times, three times a day, and within few months your sexual life will be completely changed! I promise, you'll have female ejaculations that are five feet long.

I have never met any woman with strong PC muscles who did not have orgasms; I have, however, met many with very loose PC muscles who could not achieve an orgasm. I agree that some women may have been lucky enough to be born with strong PC muscles, but the rest of you will have to work out.

Do not expect that an orgasm is something that should happen automatically or is due to you. For so many reasons, some women seem unable to have an orgasm. However, if you work on it, an orgasm is almost always achievable for women who never give up on it. Staying positive in your thoughts and attitude is most important. I have met women who have had orgasms for the first time after as long as thirty years of active sexual life. Empowering your sexual life is always a great success and feels wonderful.

Exercise for Experiencing Multi Orgasms

Is it really possible for women to reach the level of multiple orgasms? I have seen it, I have experimented, and I have witnessed it. If I had not, I could not have written this book. More than once a woman has called me to say, *"I rarely have an orgasm when I pleasure myself and have them even less often with my partner, but I am curious about Tantric massage. It seems to be interesting."* In a matter of a few sessions, such a woman will experience a complete change in her sexuality, and a big smile will appear on her face.

To achieve multiple orgasms, you will need the right cocktail of ingredients in your mind. First, you will have to trust yourself and your partner. You will need to feel chemistry with him. Both of you should have the wish to discover each other's body. All of these things may be present, but still, many women have a little voice that often says after the first orgasm, "Oh, no more, I am tired, it is enough." That voice, most of the time, is all that stops you from having multiple orgasms. That little voice should be replaced by something like, "Let's try again! Let's see what will happen." Then you should ask your partner to do something different: use manual stimulation or a different type of vibrator—whatever you feel like. Don't be discouraged if your request doesn't work the first time; try again next time!

Every journey starts with the first step, so I suggest you start by practicing the things you have read about in this chapter. After you have an orgasm, pay attention to your body. Touch your nipples, your clitoris, and your labia to feel their level of sensitivity. Observe your breathing, and get to know when your body is in the plateau phase. Then reintroduce stimulation and continue the excitation curve until you orgasm again. With practice, you will need less and less time between stages of the excitation curve, and your orgasms will flood your body.

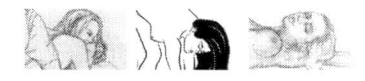

Motivational Moment

Many women are not able to experience multiple orgasms through masturbation or through sexual activities with a partner. Women have therefore often turned to Tantric massage in order to try and awaken their sexuality and experience this pleasure. By being open to the experience and to the sensations in her body, a woman may reach orgasm. This, however, is not the ultimate goal of Tantric massage, and it does not mark the end of Tantric experience. Instead, a woman should allow her partner to try and make her have an orgasm over and over again, either by manual stimulation or using vibrator. In this highly energized state, deep layers of physical and emotional tension are released, enabling many women to experience multiple orgasms. Don't be discouraged if it does not work the first time. Don't listen to your little voice saying, "Oh, no more. . . ." keep trying, and you will feel sexually pleasured and alive.

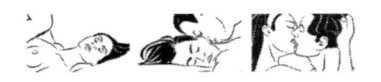

Note about Becoming a Multi Orgasmic Woman

In this chapter you have learned why some women have multiple orgasms naturally while others don't. You have read a set of suggestions and practical tips which you can apply to your sexual life in order to experience explosive, multiple orgasms that will flood your body with waves of pleasure.

Fill in the following chart to keep the record of the results of your exercises.

1. Which of these exercises did you do this week: self-pleasure, using gel enhancers, touching your nipples, your clitoris, your labia, to feel their level of sensitivity? Did you pay attention to your breathing, heartbeats, muscles contracting, and learn to know the signals your body sends when you approach the orgasm? Did you ask for what you want? Did you stimulate multiple pleasure points? Did you liberate yourself

2. What change do you want to see in yourself spiritually and sexually?

3. How do you feel about your own sexuality now you have done these exercises?

4. From 1 to 10, rate how these exercises improve the quality of your orgasms(s).

	1	2	3	4
Week 1				
Week 2				
Week 3				
Week 4				
Week 5				
Week 6				
Week 7				
Week 8				

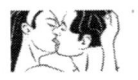

CHAPTER 10

I Lost My Sexuality! How Do I Regain It?

Los Angeles is a beautiful city to me. This is the home of movie stars. As you drive around the town you see all the beautiful faces—some famous... But, most only wishing they were famous. This is my city. It is where I belong.

On a brilliant and sunny day, I closed my eyes as I sat on my balcony overlooking the ocean. Behind me the radio was on a talk station. The program that just ended was one that I was quite fond of, dealing with current world events and the host's views on them. Unfortunately, it was followed by an arrogant conservative who takes his views to the extreme.

For a moment I dozed off, only to be awakened by one of his tirades:

"If we want the world to have any progress, we must end all nontraditional relationships," he yammered. "Random acts of sex, homosexuality, and other forms that God has told us he doesn't want! . . . ."

Turning off the radio, I decided to leave this upsetting man behind and go and check my e-mail; there was something new from a woman named Emily. Opening her e-mail, I read, "I think I have spoken to you before via email. Tell me more about your coaching session and Yoni massage. What I read online sounded amazing but almost too good to be true."

I replied, "Orgasm is 95 percent from our brains. Before we tackle that subject, I will send you some articles that I have written. Basically, the freer you become, the easier and higher your orgasm could be. This is the whole principle of your sexuality."

"What is a Tantric massage? To make it simple, it is a way to open your sensuality to make sex more enjoyable. We have a tendency to open only our genital area, but Tantric massage is a way of opening seven spiritual channels called chakras, which help us to have a better appreciation of our sexuality. Sex then becomes one long session of foreplay. Then you will always wish to receive a massage from head to toe."

In almost no time at all Emily's response came in, and I knew from experience that we were headed toward making a connection.

"I got it," Emily wrote back. But what is Tantra? Is it a sect, is it a religion. Is it from Japan or India? I am lost. Could you help me? I have gained a few pounds since my husband left me. I used to be thin, in great shape and participated in yoga regularly. I'm not entirely comfortable with my body."

"Well, ancient India had three religious traditions aimed at attaining higher cosmic consciousness and prevention of rebirth. These are the Mantra, Tantra, and Yantra," I explained to her. "Tantra means 'weave' (denoting continuity with the cosmic consciousness) in Sanskrit and involves spiritual practices and rituals that enable the practitioner to connect to the cosmic consciousness. Besides Hinduism, Tantrism has influenced the Sikh, Jain, Buddhist, and Bön religious traditions. Tantra has also influenced East Asian countries and their traditions including those of Nepal, Japan, Tibet, Burma, Korea, China, Cambodia, Mongolia, and Indonesia."

"When it spread to different countries, Tantric knowledge took different forms, but the practice of Tantra requires initiation by a teacher or guru. Once initiated, the practitioner is known as a Tantri or Tantrika.

The Tantri uses various tools such as yoga and verbalizations (mantras) or mechanical methods such as yantras to connect with the supreme consciousness like."

"*The whole subject of Tantra is interesting, but the G-spot, which is a very small part of a woman's anatomy seems to be a zone that can create lots of pleasure. The more this part of the anatomy is massaged, the more liberated and orgasmic a woman becomes. It takes time, but it is said that two years of G-spot massage could provide the same benefits as five or six years of therapy. This is only my personal experience.*"

Emily again replied immediately: "*I have had anxiety issues my entire life. I had a stomach ulcer, and I also had issues with substance abuse at a young age. I was court ordered to a state-run drug rehab program. Prior to that, I was kicked out of my mother's house at age fourteen and was sexually assaulted by a friend of the family while I was babysitting.*"

"*I have been separated from my husband for four years, so I'm a single mother of a teenage boy and a ten-year-old girl. I have not slept with anyone since my ex left to start a family with a beautiful, much younger woman. I feel so unappreciated after six years in my job. My life at the moment is quite lonely. I can't seem to love myself. Unfortunately I have not taken care of my body and am overweight. I feel my libido is gone completely. I heard you are a great coach. I need to meet you for some advice. I would like to see how this could help me feel good about myself. I wonder if I have a chance to attract your attention?*"

I was thinking, Emily not only has lost her sexuality, but her self-esteem as well.

Many women find themselves in the same situation as Emily, experiencing a loss of libido. The libido is a complex mix of ingredients, from the physical need for sex to the emotional desire to be intimate with someone. There is also a hormonal component, which varies according to the time of the month, age, gender, and many other variables.

You can easily tell if you are experiencing loss of libido by checking for these signs of diminished libido and loss of sexuality:

- You find it hard to become aroused by the same sexual stimuli that used to do the trick, and you lack the desire to be intimate with your partner.

- You feel frustrated and misunderstood by your partner, if in a committed relationship.

- When you do have sex, you experience difficulty in getting naturally lubricated, and you may experience pain during intercourse.

This chapter is for women who feel they are not reaching their full sexual potential, that they have a low sex drive, or that they feel less sensual than they did some time ago. If you feel undesirable, only get aroused with difficulty (or not at all), or feel pain (physical or emotional) when making love, this chapter is for you, too. There are several things that could lead to the "loss" of your sexuality:

Socialization and Religion: If you grew up in or are part of a very conservative and/or religious environment, it is possible that your natural need for sex (which is a basic need, along with eating, drinking, and sleeping) is well repressed or maybe even completely buried.

Trauma: If you were a victim of a sexual assault such as rape or some other type of physical abuse, your mind may be causing your body's sexual desire to decrease as a protective shield in order to prevent your exposure to more sexual experiences (which your brain now associates with pain).

Emotionally Abusive Partner: Even if you haven't been physically abused, the emotional abuse from a trusted partner is equally bad. If your partner constantly criticizes you, doesn't value your principles, and doesn't trust your choices, you accumulate frustration, which finally leads to a lack of libido.

"Dear Jean-Claude, I was molested by an older cousin for about 2 months when I was 6. There was no actual intercourse, but he made me touch his penis and French kiss him, I was just a child. Also, at the age of 15 I was date raped by my very first boyfriend. I was blacked out from something that he put in my drink, and he raped me. I was on top and managed to find my G-spot. It was quite powerful for a woman who had never had an orgasm before. I cried. I only had an orgasm with him when I was on top."

"Then I met a very sexual man, he knew a woman's body very well, and was able to push me past my own discomfort, and oh, shock, communicate to him what I liked and didn't like and what I wanted and needed sexually. Today I am reaching for your help as I feel my libido is not as powerful that it uses to be." Lisa K

I knew even the best Tantra massage will be only like a firework, then once the massage was over she will be in the dark again. We talked for many days as I nicely declined to give her a massage, and finally Lisa became aware that she was looking for love and not a Tantric massage.

Depression: In clinical depression, your thanatos (desire of death) awakens, and your eros (desire to live) is diminished. So, in the case of depression, all of the things that made you happy before are not important anymore, such as a job, a child, sexual desire. Paradoxically, the antidepressants prescribed to treat depression can also cause loss of sexual desire.

Death or Loss of a Beloved Partner: There is a natural mourning period after the loss of someone dear (either by death or separation), which lasts around six months. During this time, you feel sad, your thoughts are focused on the lost one, and you experience a loss of sexuality, fatigue, and loss of concentration.

Pregnancy or childbirth: Because of the hormonal changes a woman goes through during pregnancy, her sexual appetite may vary from being hypersexual to completely asexual. Also, after childbirth, your body produces some hormones that diminish your libido; by not encouraging you to have sex and get pregnant again right away, your body is helping you to recover from the birth and care for your newborn.

Unfortunately, Carolina was very surprised by her situation and sent me the following email, "*Dear Jean-Claude I understand, this is incredibly frustrating at times and I feel as though my body is closing in on itself. This wasn't something I predicted would happen after giving birth. It is very un-nerving to walk thru life with the ability to have multi orgasms and in the course of 9 months it's gone. But it's starting to affect my relationship. And because I know intimacy is an important aspect of any special relationship I would like to do all I can.*" I thought the words "all I can" may have a large meaning when a woman is in desperate need for a sexual pleasure.

Obesity: Here there are two possibilities. With obesity, a lack of sexuality may be psychological, as in the case of Emily, because of low self-esteem and poor self-image. Or carrying extra pounds could be blocking some hormones that normally produce the desire for sex. For example, malfunction of the thyroid, which also can lead to obesity, diminishes sex hormones as well.

Menopause: Hormones are also to blame for this cause of loss of libido. The decrease in estrogen levels that every woman experiences during menopause leads to dryness of the vagina (since less lubrication is produced), which makes intercourse painful. Also, there may be a diminished desire to have sex because, with reproductive ability gone (since egg production has stopped), the primitive brain hardly finds any reason for sex anymore.

No matter which of these situations applies to your life, you should know that there is hope and healing. In order to regain your sexuality—or to discover it, in case you were never in touch with it!—you only need four main ingredients:

- Some form of therapy: psychological (to treat or support if the cause is emotional) or medical (in case the cause is hormonal or physical).
- Time. The longer you have experienced loss of libido, the more time it could take to regain your sexuality, so be patient!
- Practice. If you have found a cause, you might have found a solution, so use it!
- Tantra. Tantra is indicated for everyone who needs to understand the body and respect and fulfill its needs, so sexual need is best discovered and increased through Tantra.

Therapy encompasses a lot of orientations and methods: art therapy, dance therapy, integrative therapy, reflex therapy, and so on. Choose the one that suits your personality and needs in order to integrate the trauma and move on.

You should remember as a general rule that emotional recovery after any traumatic event takes at least six months; the bigger the trauma, the longer the time you will need to recover emotionally. Allow your soul this time to heal.

One of the most important ingredients in recovering your sexuality is your level of confidence. If you believe that you will discover or regain your sexuality, you will do it even sooner than you expected.

Do not expect miracles when it comes to emotional and sexual recovery. As with any other parts of your body that you have not used for a long time—for example, a broken leg—your erogenous areas may have become a little numb, so you need to practice arousal in order to awaken them. Be gentle at first, and push your limits only as far as you feel comfortable and safe.

Tantra, the main ingredient in sexual recovery, is great because it treats the woman as a whole: mind, body, and spirit. Sensual massages, gentle touches, scents, and kisses combine to reintegrate your fragments and reawaken your energy.

There is no general recipe for healing yourself and regaining your sexuality. You need to listen to your body, and to your soul, step by step. Do not be afraid to cry; many women cry along this journey. Once you start the healing process, many emotions may come to the surface after years of suppression: fear, rage, sadness, revolt. Let them be, and discuss them with your therapist or express them through any form of art.

If you do not feel ready to start having sex with a partner, take small steps:

1. First, remember how your whole body feels when you touch it. Experience different kinds of touches: gentle ones with the tips of your fingers, deeper ones with the palm of your hand. Use different objects: a feather or a silk scarf for soft touches, the back of a hair brush for a more intense one. Start by touching your less sexual areas such as your hair, feet, and shoulders and

then move toward your nipples and vulva. After a few sessions of self exploring, when you feel ready, go to step 2.

2. Next, experience clitoral stimulation. Use gentle touches at first, just observing your body and your thoughts, feelings, and memories. Using a lubricant or gel enhancer could be helpful to make the experience pleasant. Take the time to explore all of your sensations, all of the positions, and all of the touches. You may need more than one try in order to climax; do not worry, this is perfectly natural. Take baby steps every time. After you have finally reached orgasm and remembered how being in touch with your sexuality feels, go one step further.

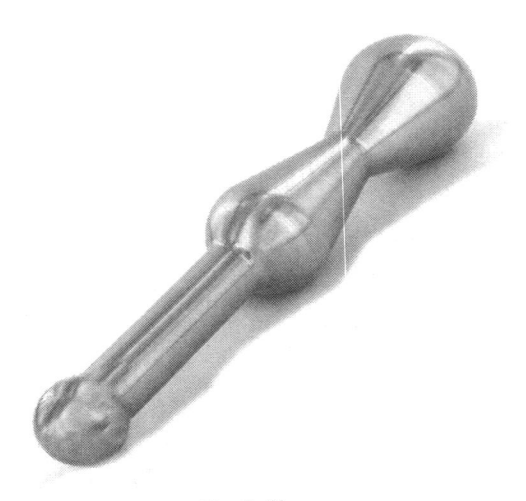

Barbells

3. Enjoy vaginal orgasms. So many women complain for good reason that they do not have vaginal orgasms, but just as often these individual women may have done little to improve their own situation. Often, it is so more easy and a usual habit to stimulate the clitoris. But to improve your sexuality takes time, and you should view that time as an investment. Even if you

were not able previously to reach vaginal orgasm, try again now, with your energy reawakened and your sexuality regained. Read the section about Kegel exercises (Chapter 7), and start doing them every day. In order to experience a vaginal orgasm, your PC muscles must be in good shape. Try to squeeze around a bar (a barbell made for this purpose, buy one on line). (*see picture of Barbell dildo*) The weight of the object will help to isolate your vaginal muscles, which is the most effective way to do this exercise. Use a lot of water-based lubricant, and when you are sufficiently aroused, experiment with the speed and trajectory of your fingers. Try out different positions: on your back, on your belly, kneeling with your legs apart. After exploring your vagina and the sensations you have when fingering, if you are comfortable, use a dildo or a vibrator. Again, do not use the lubricant sparingly: Use plenty! Try out various positions to experience different angles of penetration. This will help you find your G-spot or A-spot, which in time will give you great pleasure. When you are sufficiently wet, start squeezing and releasing your PC muscles as you guide the vibrator in and out of your vagina. At that point you will start to feel the orgasm. Again, first you build up your vaginal muscle practicing your Kegel exercises, 100 times a day. Second you will use a dildo or a vibrator and your vagina will squeeze it and release it many times imagining the penis of your lover until you feel that orgasm coming up and giving you pleasure. You will need to play around with your vibrator to find the right spot. Third, you have now plenty of practices and can start to build up to that orgasm where you will replace your vibrator by the penis of your partner the same way that you have use a vibrator. Don't be afraid to ask your partner to slow down, the vaginal penetration has to be done slowly - very slowly; your muscles will squeeze around his penis. Don't worry, he will love it. Some women do not like vibrators, so you may use any short steel bar or the handle of a hairbrush. At first, use your aid slowly, and then speed up the rhythm. Remember, you dictate the rhythm, the moves your hips make, and your position. With a little practice, you will be able to use one hand on the vibrator and the other to stimulate your clitoris.

Over time and with practice, you will be able to use these techniques with the penis of your partner, and you will not feel exposed or vulnerable or inadequate any more. You will live your sexuality to its full capacity, love your body, engage in emotional and sexual connection to your partner(s), and simply feel happy and fulfilled.

This is all about: to build up the muscles of the vagina, then to find the right spot for you to have an orgasm. Don't forget practice, practice, practice …and enjoy

What Else Can I do To Regain My Sexuality?

The most important part of the process of regaining your sexuality is not finding a solution but finding the cause. Why? Because once you have found the specific cause (or combination of causes) that applies to you, your solution is right there in front of you. You just need to re-arrange the letters, so to speak.

- **Obesity**. If you have come to the conclusion that you do not feel sexy anymore, and that your weight is affecting your self-esteem and your ability to enjoy your sexual life, you have the answer: Lose some weight. Although it seems terribly difficult at first (you might be just like Emily, who was a single mom, sexually and emotionally frustrated from her last relationship, and always busy and stressed out), once you set your mind to it, you can start a diet plan (consider consulting a nutritionist), start to exercise, and in no time, you will be back to your twenty-year-old figure.

- **Depression or the loss of a partner.** For depression, psychotherapy as well as medical treatment can be helpful. If your antidepressant make you sleepy and diminishes your libido, speak to your doctor to have your medication adjusted. Tantra is a great way to get back in touch with your body and to start to care again about the way it feels, the way it looks, and what it needs. Meditation and yoga are two other great methods to help with depression.

- **Physical or emotional trauma.** Psychotherapy is also very useful for this cause of diminished libido—along with some form of contact sport (boxing, martial arts), which does wonders for repressed aggressiveness.

- **Menopause.** Many doctors and scientists have tried to find some form of medical treatment that will make "forever young" stories come true, at least regarding the sex part. Because the main cause of loss of sexuality during menopause is the low production of estrogen, the pharmaceuticals companies came up with estrogen supplements for women in menopause. Their main effect is an increased vaginal lubrication, which makes the intercourse more pleasant. However, no medicine can trick your brain into thinking you are still very young; the only way to make your brain believe it, is if you actually do believe that you're young. Sounds complicated? It isn't. Just do the things that make you happy: Be active, go out, find a hobby, travel, go dancing, and you will see that, along with your joy in life, you will also recover your sexuality. Some women even find that they have more intense orgasms after menopause than before. My mother had sex until her late eighties, so it is possible! Sexuality is a state of mind. Genetics can play a role, but ultimately your sexuality is mostly about what you decide or feel in your mind.

Because every journey starts with the first step, you can try a few of the next exercises to help you regain your sexuality. You can try them no matter what the specific cause of your loss of libido may be, because they are meant to open your heart and improve your self-esteem—two things that no person has too much of.

Exercises for Regaining Your Sexuality

- Start writing erotic short stories or paint erotic scenes. At first you may find the stories boring and not arousing, but keep trying. Let yourself write whatever fantasies come through your head.

- Smile at the beginning and later begin to flirt with cute strangers in public. You do not have to go further; just flirt with them and have fun.

- Wear lacy, sexy, transparent underwear. It is not necessary to be in a relationship; wear it for yourself, and pay attention to the way it makes you feel.

- Undress and take nude pictures of yourself. Pose for the camera. If you have a partner, pretend to be a nude supermodel, and let him take pictures of you.

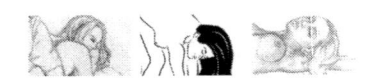

Motivational Moment

Do you want to feel free? To experience pleasure and explore your sensuality? Do you want to feel desire, lust, pure sexual passion? Do you want your body to feel whole? To abandon yourself in your partner's arms and enjoy your sexual union? If you answered with a loud "Yes!" to at least one of these questions, this chapter is for you and about you. Read it carefully, and apply the tips to your life. Learn how to move on, and feel the joy of exploring your sexuality.

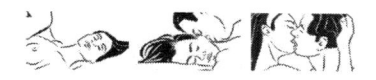

Note about Regaining Your Sexuality

This is a chapter for women who are survivors, who have been through traumas and not only outlived the nightmare but found that they still have the inner resources to learn more about their bodies. This chapter is for women to remember what pleasure feels like and what to do to experience it again; to regain their sexuality; to feel happy and completed.

Fill out this log to keep a record of the results of your exercises:

1. Which of these exercises to regain sexuality did you do this week? Did you self-explore your body with a feather or a silk scarf? Gently caress your clitoris? Did you introduce a finger or two into your vagina? Did you feel your G-spot or your A-spot and start exercising your PC muscles using a barbell or vibrator? Did you lose weight? Meet a new lover? Increase your self-esteem? Go on vacation with your husband? Did you write erotic short stories? Did you start to smile and begin to flirt with people you met? Did you wear lacy, sexy, transparent underwear? Did you undress and take nude pictures of yourself?

2. What change do you want to see in yourself, spiritually and sexually?

3. How do you feel about your own sexuality now that you have done these exercises?

4. On a scale of 1 to 10, with 10 the maximum, how have these exercises improved the quality of your orgasm(s)?

	1	2	3	4
Week 1				
Week 2				
Week 3				
Week 4				
Week 5				
Week 6				
Week 7				
Week 8				

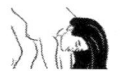

CHAPTER 11

The Tantric Lingam: Anatomy and Pleasuring of the Penis and Male G-spot

The practice of Tantra deals with channeling energy as well as pleasure. Interestingly enough, the Sanskrit word for the male organ or penis, *lingam*, loosely translates to mean "wand of light." I find this immensely attention-grabbing as one of the reasons why we seek to channel energy and pleasure is to enlighten individuals. Before we look at some Tantric practices that allow a lover to pay passionate homage to the lingam, let's start with a small anatomy lesson.

The penis, of course, is the organ though which semen passes when a man has an orgasm, and the male also passes urine through his penis. The penis has six thousand nerve endings. No wonder a female orgasm is more pleasurable than the male orgasm—the clitoris has 9000 nerves! (*see drawing; The penis, of course, is the organ though which semen passes when a man has an orgasm*)

The penis engorges when it erects, which is what happens when a man is sexually excited. The penis is made of many cavernous membranes, and these fill with blood during erection. The rushing blood can make the entire penis throb in time to a man's heartbeat. Erection is caused by a number of physical factors and also by psychic stimulation. For instance, men often use fantasies to cause or maintain an erection.

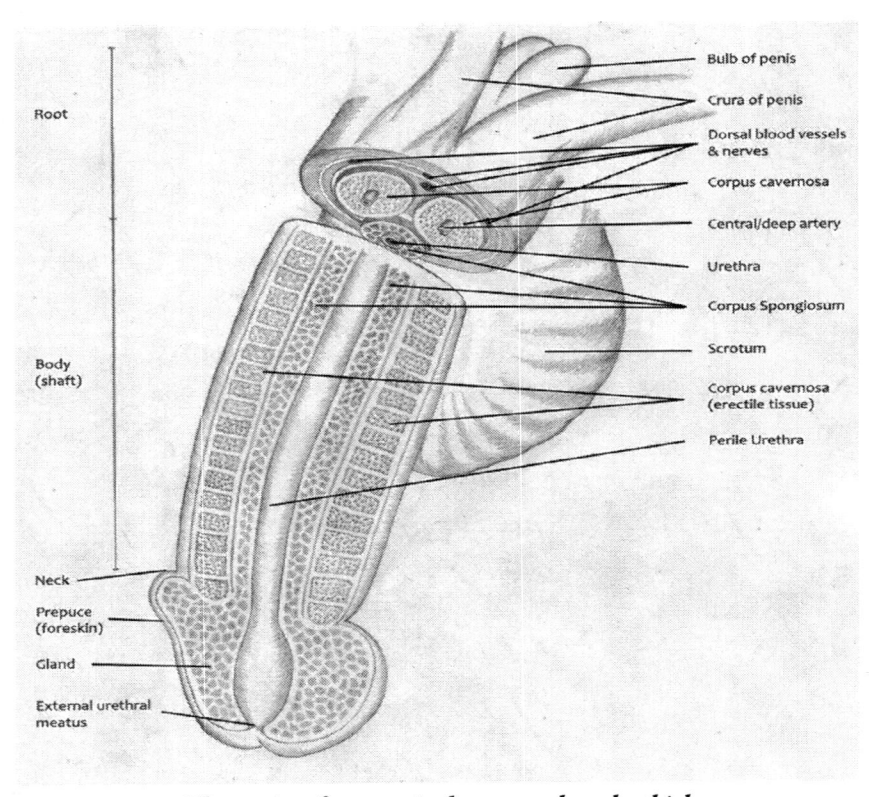

The penis, of course, is the organ though which semen passes when a man has an orgasm

Some men are circumcised while others are not. Circumcision is usually performed on male babies, and the debate as to whether circumcision is better for health or not is ongoing. Many men are satisfied with their parents decision to have their penis circumcised, but many other men feel they are missing a great amount of pleasure. Today major medical societies in western countries do not recommend circumcision but leave that choice to the parents. The origin of the circumcision is uncertain. It may have been for hygiene reason, or a symbol of the transition age from enfant to warrior, or to show a woman her mate could handle a great amount of pain, or refrain the male from masturbation practice. However, circumcision is also an indication of the religious beliefs of a male baby's parents. If uncircumcised, the penis will have a fleshy covering at the tip called the foreskin, which needs to be pulled back to uncover the head. Excitement often is measured by the hardness of the penis; however, a man may be very turned on without his penis being hard, and vice-versa.

The perinea—the area between the anus and the testicles (contained within the scrotum)—and the scrotum itself are filled with nerve endings, as is the anal area. Understanding how a man's sexual anatomy corresponds to female anatomy is useful to both sexes in Tantric lovemaking and massage:

- Head of penis = Clitoris
- Foreskin = Hood
- Scrotum = Labia Majora
- Shaft = Labia Minora
- Testicles = Ovaries
- Perinea = Perinea
- Anus = Anus.

Pleasuring the Lingam

Setting the mood for pleasure is often important. The female wishing to please her man may use candles, play soft music in the background, and even perform a sensual dance just for him.

In Tantric lingam sex, the female, wishing to build trust and intimacy with her partner, begins by massaging the male on the

- Chest
- Nipples
- Thighs
- Abdomen
- Inner thigh.

Anticipation is as important as touch in the beginning of this wondrous adventure. Before starting, he will have emptied his bowels and bladder, and you will have bathed together, making sure that you are both as fresh as possible. Remember again to build anticipation.

The most sensitive area of the lingam itself is just under the head, a spot that is called the frenulum. This is the slight indentation that you will see on one side of the head (glans) of the lingam and continuing on its underside. You will always know that this is your lover's most sensitive spot as he may jump or moan when you touch it.

Pleasuring the Lingam Manually

Massage lubrication onto his lingam, and then wrap your hand around his member, moving your fist up and down. Change the speed as well as the pressure as you move past the corona and the frenulum. The male orgasm is different than a woman orgasm. It starts to go to a very high level rapidly and also go down rapidly. (*see diagram: The male orgasm is different than a woman orgasm. It goes to a very high level rapidly and goes down also rapidly*) Here are some more ideas for touching the lingam:

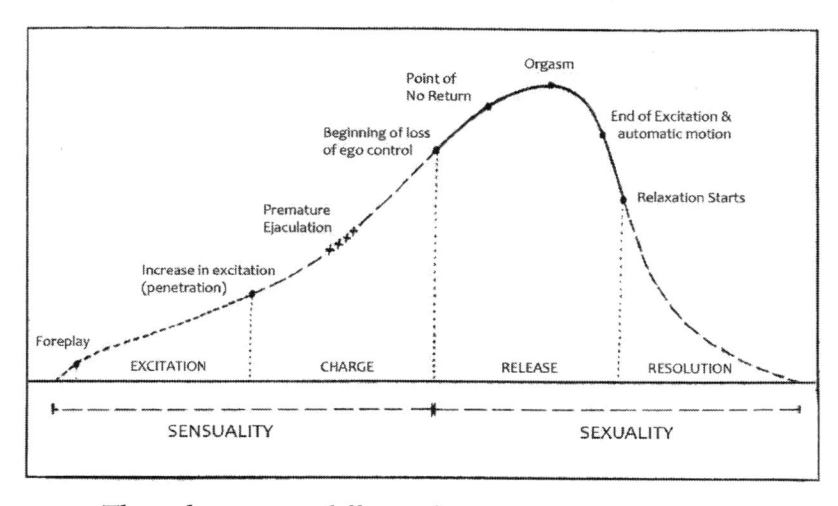

The male orgasm is different than a woman orgasm. It goes to a very high level rapidly and goes down also rapidly

- Use both hands.
- Make the ring of your fingers rather tight.
- Then loosen them.
- Use your other hand to fondle his testicles.
- Roll the lingam between your palms.
- Move your hands in opposite directions.
- Make a twisting motion.
- Increase speed near orgasm.

Above all let him know what a turn on it is for you to give him pleasure like this!

Make sure that you do the following:

- Start slowly.
- Use enthusiasm.

- Praise him.
- Don't stop, even after ejaculation, so that you do not lose the mood.

The Ultimate Pleasure

Fellatio brings pleasure to a man's lingam with mouth, tongue, and lips. Many women have told me that their men say that the moans and groans elicited from them by fellatio made them finally understand what oral sex must feel like to a woman. Women thus should understand why men love fellatio so much!

Many women do not wish to take part in fellatio, yet they are very happy when their men perform oral sex on them. Just remember that when someone is being selfish in a relationship, something will cease to work. Remember also, ladies, that when you perform fellatio on your man, you are also educating him about a way he can give you the ultimate pleasure.

Some women, unfortunately, have had negative childhood experiences that may make them reticent about giving fellatio to their lovers, which is understandable. Tantra may help these situations.

Getting Started with Fellatio

To begin with fellatio, make sure he's relaxed. The 69 position is excellent! Start slowly and

- Touch him with your hands.
- Use kisses.
- Add licks.

- Bring the lingam wholly into your mouth.

Approach

If you maintain a smile and appear to love what you are doing, this will help. Attitude is reflected in how you touch and lick him. Make it something that you look forward to!

Emotions transfer from you to him. Thus if you are truly loving, your partner will feel even more relaxed and satisfied, and this will guide him to an unbelievable orgasm. A man can actually see in his woman's eyes that she loves giving him this much pleasure. Some men describe oral sex as being inflamed with passion!

Men love fellatio because it strokes their egos. It makes them feel out of the ordinary, significant, appreciated, and intensely satisfied. It will encourage him to be loyal and to have a greater desire to pleasure you in return.

Intersperse your actions during fellatio with comments that let him know that you love doing it and that it's turning you on. Tell him how fantastic he tastes. Men love the element of surprise, so use your hottest fellatio tips when least expected. He will not develop the desire to look for someone else. Oral sex will strengthen your relationship and bring you ever closer to your lover.

Fellatio Step by Step

- Lick his lingam, wetting your tongue frequently.
- Cover your teeth with your lips.
- Smile.
- Note his feedback (moans, breathing, and body movements).

The Meatus

The meatus is the urethral opening, which has a tremendous amount of sensory nerves. Run your tongue over it, either flat or pointed.

Suction Strength

A certain amount of suction is welcomed as it compresses the lips onto the teeth and creates a cavern with the inside of your cheeks that caresses the lingam all over. Too much suction or for too long a time is not so pleasant.

Deep Throat

To practice, use your fingers or a spoon. It's all a matter of mind over matter, and it will matter! If you know how to contain your gag reflex, much can be said for a "Deep Throat" entry, which allows you to massage the lingam while it is in your throat. A kind of swallowing maneuver is recommended; however, depending on the sensitivity of his lingam, this may hasten ejaculation. Also, you may caress the scrotum with your tongue while you hold his lingam deep in your throat.

Be sure and use your hands as well, to give your mouth a rest, or to prevent entry too deeply into your throat if you have not yet mastered your gag reflex. Keeping your eyes open and making eye contact is excellent.

Perinea

The perinea has sensitive nerve endings that cause the head of the lingam to swell. Pressing on the perinea with two fingers may heighten ejaculation as it is linked to the man's prostate. Some women prefer to use their tongue to press on the perinea.

The Testicles

It's fine to pause and move from the lingam to pay attention to the testicles.

- Lick them individually.
- Suck one into your mouth.
- Run your tongue along both.
- Suck both in and tongue them. (*see drawing: Suck both in and tongue them*)

Delaying Ejaculation

To control ejaculation during fellatio, grasp the lingam with your forefinger wrapped above the top of the shaft close to the base. Have your mate signal you prior to ejaculation, and then use your thumb to compress his urethra. This will hold back the ejaculate so you can continue pleasuring him.

Mental Rush

Once ejaculation happens, the mental rush from fellatio is incomparable. This will bring unparalleled trust and intimacy to your relationship. Both the receiver and the giver will have felt tremendous pleasure. The female becomes irresistible to the male, especially when she swallows his gift and smiles to show her man her empty mouth.

Why Swallow?

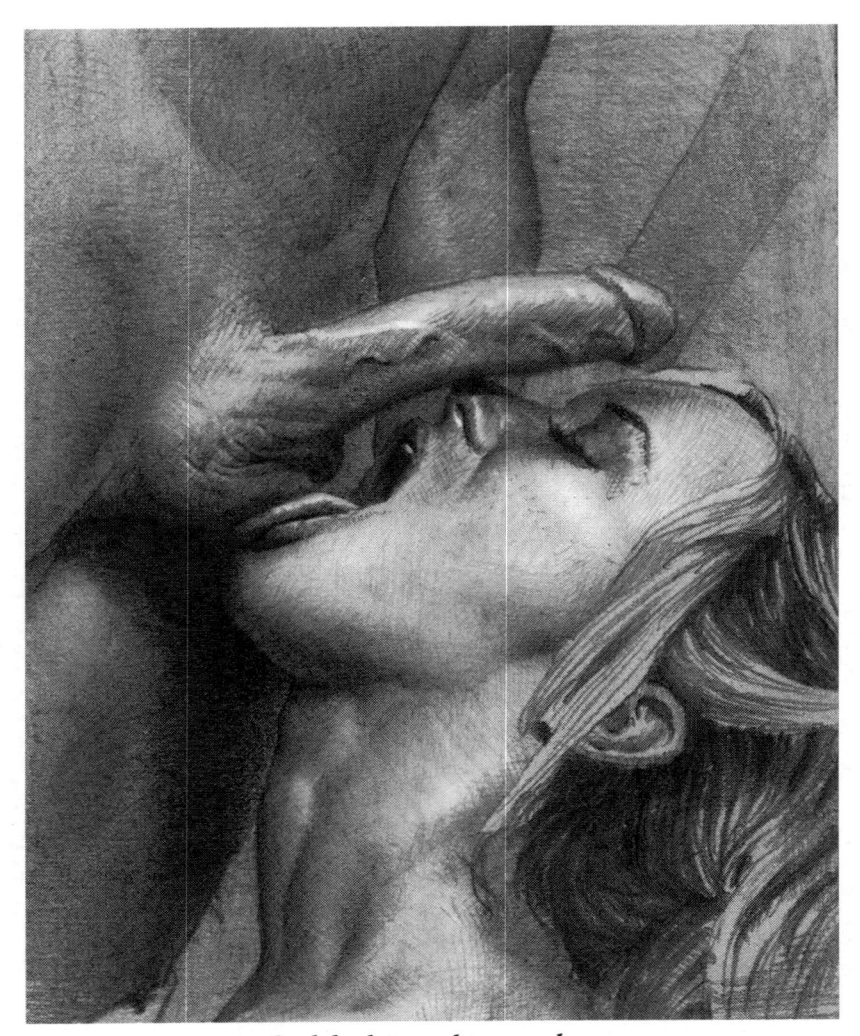

Suck both in and tongue them

You would feel hurt if he

- spit out your secretions,
- hurried to the bathroom,

- used mouthwash,
- brushed his teeth.

Swallowing his ejaculate will bring

- Unconditional acceptance.
- Feelings of love.
- The chance to keep romancing his body.
- Emotional satisfaction.
- Health and wellness, since the fluid is composed of protein.

Some women love the taste! And some men feel even closer to their lover if the woman reserves some cum in her mouth, and allows him to share the cum with her as they kiss. Some feel that this is the definitive act of intimacy between lovers. Men also love to cum in a woman's mouth because it is taboo and "naughty."

Fellatio with the Uncircumcised

American men are generally circumcised; the figure is about 60 percent, whereas worldwide it is about 15 percent. When performing fellatio on an uncircumcised male, there can be pain if the foreskin is yanked back too quickly or if a tooth accidentally rubs against and snags it. Therefore, be extra gentle with your uncircumcised partner. You might try to encircle the area within the foreskin with your tongue.

Some women prefer uncircumcised men, and others prefer circumcised. With circumcision, there is less chance of bad smells, off tastes, or any other offensiveness due to even a trivial amount of uncleanliness. Also, circumcision helps to prevent many diseases, but the final word on the practice has not yet come through from medical authorities.

Those who prefer their men uncut say that the head of the lingam is much more sensitive when the foreskin is intact.

Deep-Throating a Long Lingam

Long swords go down a sword swallower's throat, so with fellatio, accepting a longer lingam is just a matter of setting your mind. Start slow, but when you are ready, open your throat even more while taking in the lingam. Next, swallow hard to make your tongue move inward, and at the same time, push your head forward. Then just do this over and over again, adding new depth to his pleasure.

Irrumatio

Basically, irrumatio is fellatio with a change of position. Fellatio lends control to the woman, allowing her to move her mouth, lips, and tongue, but irrumatio simply gives the control to the man, the one being fellated. While the woman lies on the mattress, perhaps with her head hanging off the bed, it is the male who then moves his lingam in and out of her mouth. Pompeiian frescoes testify that irrumatio was a highly favored Roman sexual act. Part of the joy of irrumatio, for the male, is being able to watch his lingam slide into the throat of his lover and admiring the bulge that he is obviously creating.

Assorted Hints

There are so many ways to make fellatio even more exciting. For instance,

- Use a mentholated candy drop to create tingles.
- Use ice as a cool tool for stimulation.

- Alternate ice with hot tea or coffee for extra stimulation.
- Humming while giving fellatio imparts excitement.
- Rubbing the head of the lingam on your face as well as your lips gives a different sensation.
- Press the lingam into your palate using the very back of your tongue and then release—and do it again and again!

Positioning and Locations

- Place pillows behind the male.
- Sit, kneel, or lie down between his bent legs.
- Once he's relaxed, focus on erogenous zones.
- Save the lingam for last.
- Gently massage the lingam.
- Move around in your home.
- Try the shower, too.
- Go for a drive.
- Do it in the kitchen.
- Do it in any secluded place.
- Use surprise locales.

Lingam Exercise

It is important to learn each and every nuance of fellatio prior to performing it on your mate. Thus you may wish to practice the gentle art of fellatio on a banana, a great way to start! Or you might turn an ice cream cone into an erotic show for your mate, which will be greatly appreciated. When it comes to actually doing it, fellatio is a passionate exercise.

Motivational Moment

Men are notorious for having fantasies, and satisfying those fantasies will bring you both much closer together. The trust and intimacy that come from fellatio will surprise you. Fellatio is one of the greatest pleasures that you can give to a man, so you will want to be good at it. Men fall in love with the woman who enjoys giving good fellatio. It means a lot if you turn it into the wildest experience that you can!

So many emotions can be attributed to the act of fellatio: joy, physical happiness, caring from your partner, and the trust that is instilled. Wishing to give a man so much pleasure involves compassion. Fellatio will cement a relationship, for it brings contentment and, of course, eventually the ultimate satisfaction.

Part of the excitement of fellatio is the power that a woman feels when performing it. She feels the lingam grow in her mouth and knows that she alone is responsible for that growth. She thinks, "Those are my kisses, my tongue, my mouth, and my dedication to him that are causing that arousal!". A woman also enjoys being told by her lover that she is the best with this sexual art.

The Male G-Spot

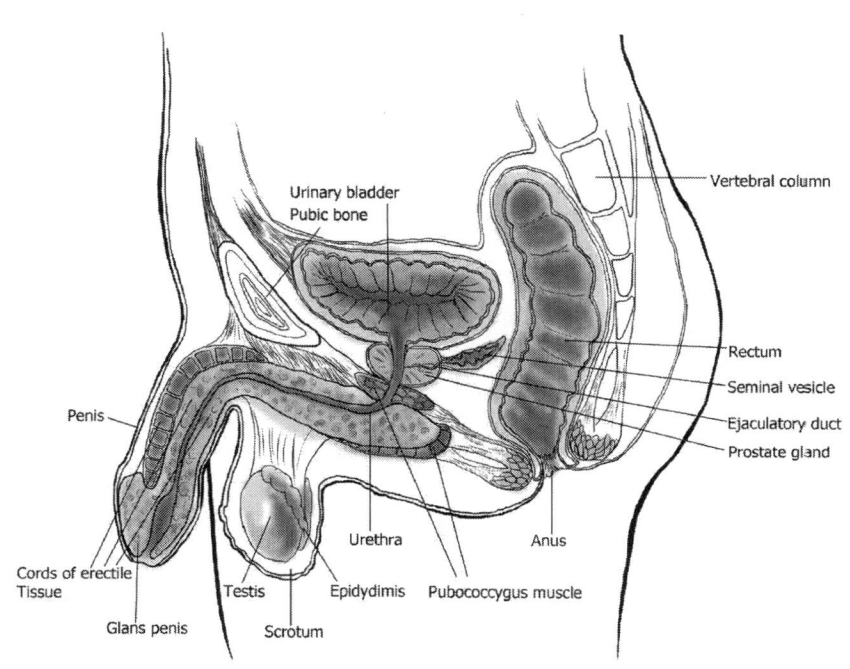

The prostate would rarely be referred to as a "male G-spot

The male's prostate corresponds to the woman's G-spot. Chemically, the liquid produced by the prostate to carry sperm and the liquid expelled during female ejaculation are virtually identical. Medically speaking, the prostate would rarely be referred to as a "male G-spot"; this is more along the lines of an understanding between lovers. (*see drawing: The prostate would rarely be referred to as a "male G-spot*)

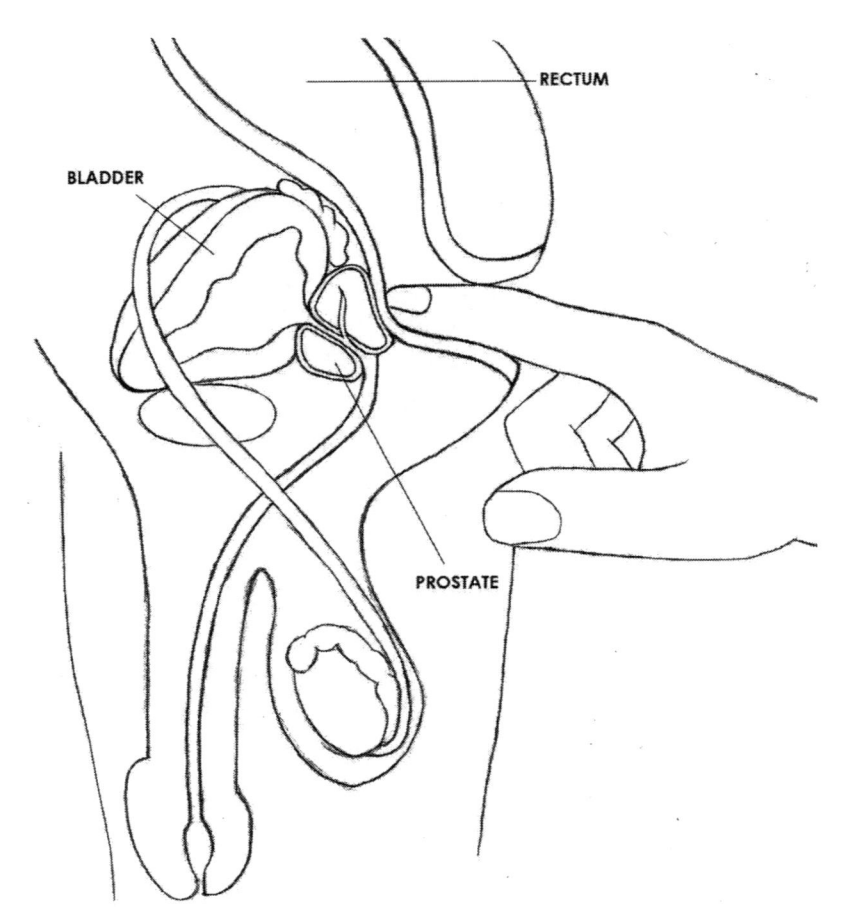

Prostate Milking

By massaging the prostate, seminal (prostate) fluid may be squeezed out or "milked."

Found in both Asia and the Far East in drawings and documents, prostate milking goes back thousands of years. By massaging the prostate, seminal (prostate) fluid may be squeezed out or "milked." This helps to keep the gland healthy, helping to prevent prostate problems as the man ages. Medically, milking will cleanse or detoxify the prostate, so it not only feels wonderful but can have positive health benefits as well.

(*see drawing: By massaging the prostate, seminal (prostate) fluid may be squeezed out or "milked."*)

Position

Some men may be squeamish about having you enter their anal area. You should discuss what is to happen, and he should void both urine and feces. You can take a relaxing hot shower together as well.

You should make the experience as sensuous as possible. Start, for example, by doing some sensuous touching, kissing, licking, and massaging of the anal area as the anus is a very erogenous zone. Tell him that you wish to try this as you've heard that it will give him a highly intense release, and that this Tantric method is said to bring a man multiple orgasms!

When you're both ready to try the milking, he should lie down on his back with his legs bent at the knees. You may use a rubber glove, a condom, or your bare fingers, provided your nails are short.

You reach his gland through his anus, and you will find it approximately half a finger's length inside of him. Use liberal amounts of high quality water-based lubricant. Tease his anus lightly, and continue to stimulate his lingam with your other hand or mouth (*see drawing: By massaging the prostate, seminal (prostate) fluid may be squeezed out or "milked."*).

Location of the Prostate

Since he is on his back, once you have inserted your finger into his anus, you may begin to look for the prostate by curling your finger upward toward his belly. It is a tiny bump, probably about two inches into his anus. It is about the size of a walnut and may be softer in the middle.

You will want to carefully press upward while massaging in a circular manner. Most men also enjoy a "come here" motion with your finger. Above all, both partners should be ultra relaxed and proceed unhurriedly and tenderly. It is suggested that you slightly vary the pressure you use. Keep in mind that just as you have a special technique you especially enjoy with your own G-spot, your partner will be the same—but keep in mind that you will not need to massage as vigorously as he might massage your own G-spot. As this is very sensual, there should be an erection involved, but if not, you can combine this with pleasing him orally. The man should breathe deeply, relax, and enjoy the massage.

Result

For many males, milking the prostate causes them to experience ejaculation almost immediately. Few can put off the inevitable, so if you find that he is enjoying it tremendously, you may wish to stop the massage for a bit to allow him to retain control over his ejaculation, and then resume.

Male G-Spot Exercise

Discuss prostate massage thoroughly with your mate. Be sure to press the point about how interested you are and how you would love to see him have an utterly blissful experience.

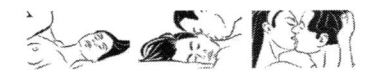

Motivational Moment

For yourself, the rich warm feelings you will get in sharing this with your mate are extremely gratifying! This is also a way of making sure that your partner's prostate is behaving normally, i.e., causing him to ejaculate rapidly. In addition, regular prostate massage may aid erectile problems.

Penetration

Men, I will share a secret with you: The key to give a woman the ultimate pleasure, both in Tantric massage and lovemaking, is TEASING. *You have to build up the pleasure by creating expectation for your partner.* When you are making love, do not focus primarily on having an orgasm and "getting it over with."

- Put all of your energy, imagination, and self-control into teasing your partner and increasing her level of desire. Start using these techniques during foreplay. Tease her when you kiss her, and when you touch her. When kissing her lips, get closer to her, open your mouth a little, let her feel your breath, and then gently touch her lips with your tongue, and pull away.

- Do the same when touching her breasts: Caress their outline, kiss their soft skin, get closer to the nipple, but do not touch it. Let her imagine that you will, but do not give it to her right away. This way, her desire will grow more and more.

- When you are both ready for penetration, put your lingam on her vulva, and tap it a little. Rub it on her clitoris, through her labia, and on the perinea. She will start moving her hips and breathing faster and maybe will even ask you to get inside her. Use your self-control to resist her pleas, and tease her more.

242 Sex: Woman First

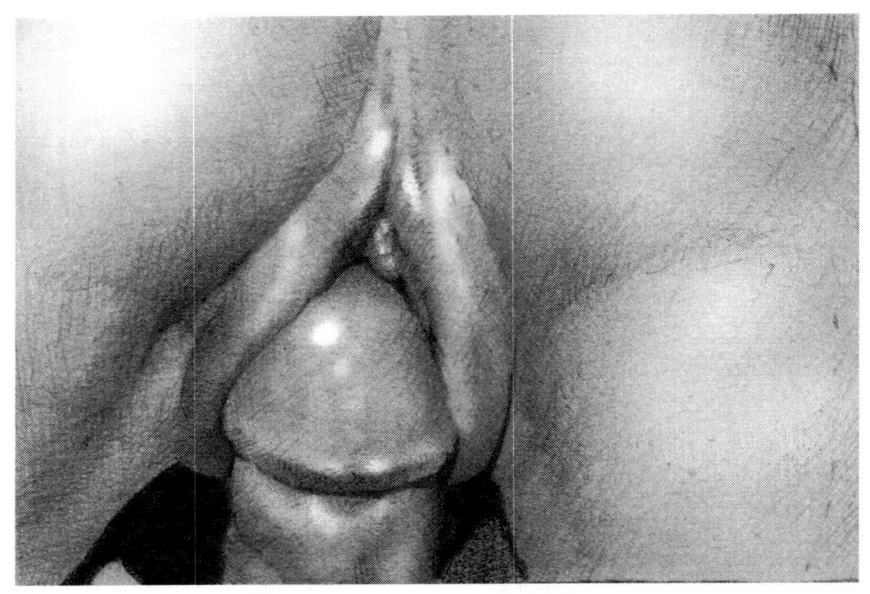

The penetration includes the in-and-out motion should be done extremely SLOOOWLY

- When she is close to orgasm, then you may start to penetrate her, but not all at once. First, insert the top of your penis, only the top, use an in-and-out motion, and let her feel the pleasure. This will allow desire to grow stronger for you both. Next, insert more and more of your penis, inch by inch. The penetration includes the in-and-out motion and should be done extremely SLOOOWLY. (*see drawing: The penetration includes the in-and-out motion should be done extremely SLOOOWLY*) When your Goddess realizes that you are slowly moving out, she may feel that you are going to leave her in that arousal. She will beg for you to faster. But you are in complete control. She is begging you, you are driving her nicely insane. For you to reach the deepness of her vagina, it should take at least 15 minutes, more if you can. Take all your time to have your whole penis introduced in her vagina and take more time to slowly getting in and out. You can keep doing for hours and hours. More time equal more pleasure for your Goddess. Remember the slower you go and the more you are getting in control of your ejaculation, she will realize that you have a very powerful mind, and she will let go and enjoy the best penetration she ever had. With every inch, her pleasure will grow, and she will be ever closer to an explosive orgasm.

- After her first orgasm, if you can still go on, do not stop. This way, she will experience multiple orgasms, each one growing in intensity and coming up faster than the previous one. This is called "riding the wave," and it will offer both you and your Goddess an incredible sexual experience.

- Women: you should enjoy deeply that practice by focusing on your pleasure only. Women: you must focus on your vagina only and meditate on the extreme pleasure of the penis entering and penetrating extremely slowly; feeling like your whole body has been taken over by your God. Your PC muscles will now enter in action with plenty of time to squeeze the penis which is penetrating your vagina. Squeeze and relax the penis, push your muscles like you learn during your Kegel exercises, then you will feel your first vaginal orgasm. If you never had a vaginal orgasm, it will take some practice but you have your whole life to reach that beautiful state of vaginal orgasm. The difference between you and the one, who always have a vaginal orgasm, is that she does it naturally. You will have to practice a little bit more than the other, then it will come naturally for you too.

Note about the Lingam, Male G-spot, and Penetration

As you read this chapter, you have learned about the most sensitive portions of your lover's physical makeup, but you have also learned more about the mental side of your lover with relation to his lingam. Some men say that fellatio is actually that "Love Potion #9"!

This chapter has illuminated an additional manner by which you may bring your partner tremendous joy. The prostate is easy to find, and once he has felt the pleasure of male G-spot massage, he will probably ask for it again and again.

By continuing with the exercises, you have both experienced improvement in the art of lovemaking.

Fill in this log to record the results of your exercises:

1. Which of these Tantric lingam exercises did you do this week: Did you massage his penis manually? Did you practice orally on him? Did you massage his prostate? Did you do Deep Throat? Did he penetrate you very slowly with in-and-out motions?

2. What change do you want to see in yourself spiritually and sexually?

3. How do you feel about your own sexuality now that you have done these exercises?

4. On a scale of 1 to 10, with 10 the maximum, how have these exercises improved the quality of your orgasm(s)?

	1	2	3	4
Week 1				
Week 2				
Week 3				
Week 4				
Week 5				
Week 6				
Week 7				
Week 8				

CHAPTER 12

The Best Six Sex Positions for a Woman to Achieve Orgasm

Everyone has their favorites, of course, many achieve an orgasm when her God is on top and her clitoris is stimulated against his body. But the six best sex positions from the point of view of this book are the ones that either create great G-spot stimulation or better clitoral stimulation. As you will see, each of the following was designed with one or the other in mind, but take into account that the key to it all is to breathe deeply together.

The Surprise

With yourself on all fours, your lover stands behind you as he enters you. This is sometimes called "Congress of the Dog" in the philosophy of the *Kama Sutra*. As he bends toward you, he may use both hands to romance your clitoris, or one hand for your clitoris and the other for your breast. His lingam will pierce you in such a way as to naturally stimulate your G-spot as well as make deep penetration. Thrusting may be done by either the male or the female, or they may both grind against each other. (*see drawing: The surprise*)

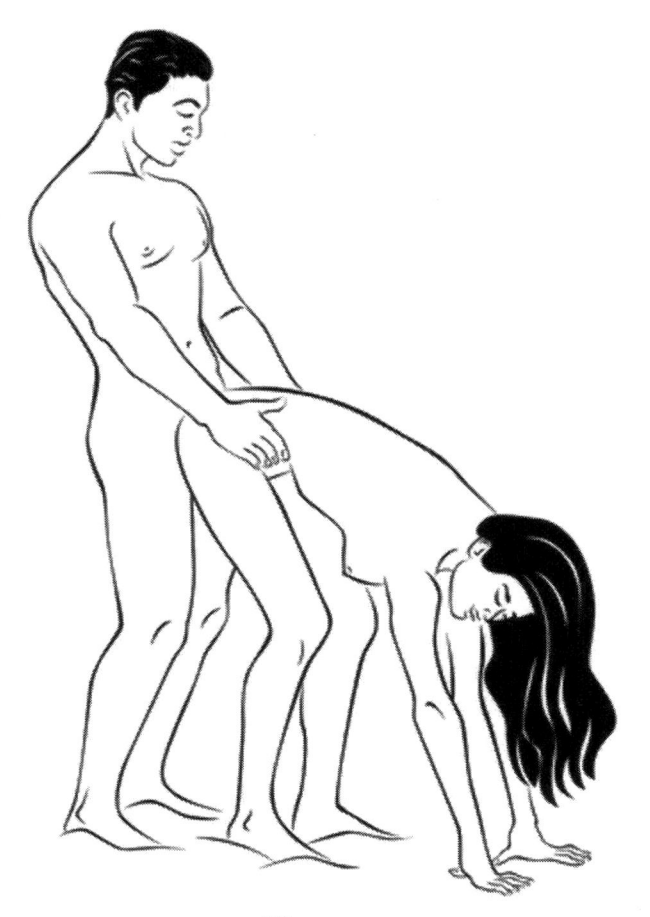

The surprise

The Organ Grinder

While you are on your back, your partner enters you, and then you bring your knees to your chest as he supports himself on his arms. You can hook your ankles over his shoulders if you desire. His lingam will be romancing both your G-spot and your A-spot in the deeper recesses of your yoni. This position is even mentioned in the *Kama Sutra*, where it is called "The Germinated Seed." (*see drawing: The Organ Grinder*)

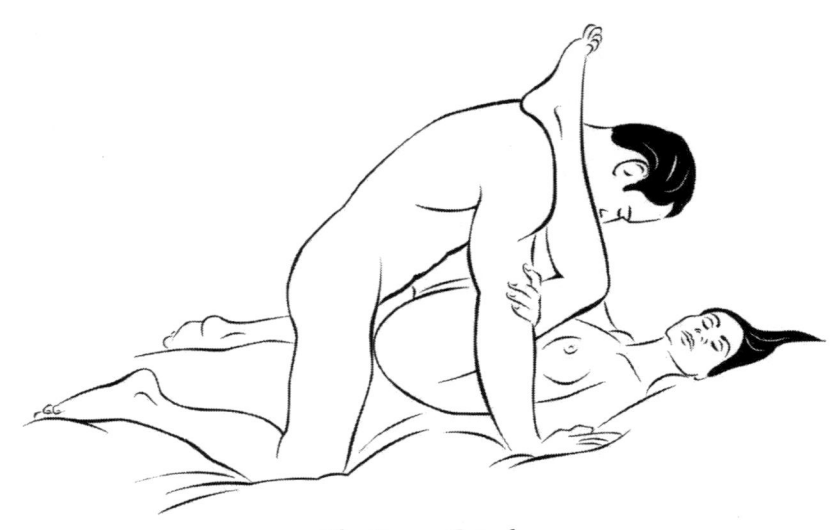

The Organ Grinder

The Yab Yum

This position is excellent for building up sexual energy. With your partner seated, place yourself on your man's lap with your legs around his torso. Pelvic rocking movements are done together, and you will both be able to practice simultaneous breathing to allow you to ride the wave. This blissful position, sometimes referred to as the Kama Sutra position, gives deep access and keeps your hands free to romance each other, he by stroking your clitoris as well as your G-spot. (*see drawing: The Yab Yum*)

Deep Impact

While lying on your back on a bed, sofa, or armchair, your partner kneels in front of you on the floor. Your vagina is at the same level of his penis. For more support while moving, rest your legs over his shoulders. Your hands are free to caress him or yourself, and your partner can use his hands to stimulate your breast or clitoris. The name of the position is no coincidence, as this position facilitates a deeper penetration, allowing your partner to enter you completely. Your partner could use a pillow under his knees to increase his height and comfort. (*see drawing: Deep Impact*)

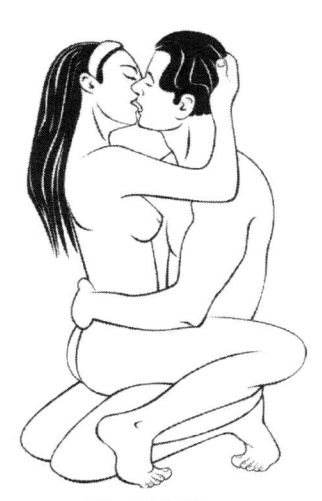

The Yab Yum

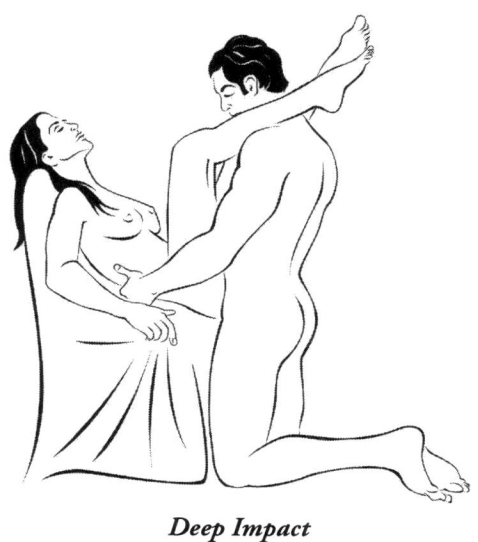

Deep Impact

Doggy Style

This is a well-known position. With you supporting yourself on knees and hands, your partner penetrates you from behind while also sitting on his knees. Try this position on a steady couch or on the floor to increase stability and allow for more intense movement. Your partner can use his hands to stimulate your clitoris or breasts. As with most back positions, penetration is deeper and stimulation of the G-spot is stronger. (*see drawing: Doggy Style*)

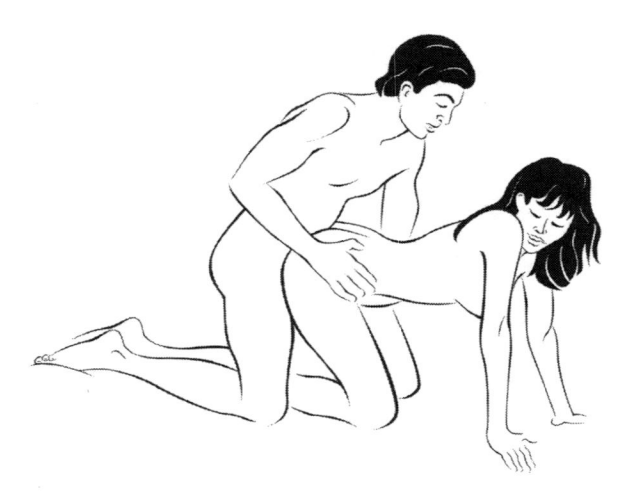

Doggy Style

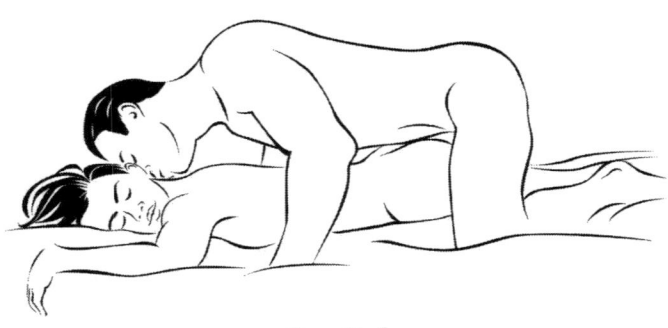

Deer Style

Deer Style

While you lie on your stomach, your partner penetrates you from behind. Spread your legs and push your buttocks up for easier access. You could stay like this, with your partner lying on top of you with his chest on your back and his legs closed, or you could close your legs and let him keep his legs on the outside. During penetration, your partner can rest on his elbows and use his hands to fondle your breast, or you could stimulate your clitoris. (*see drawing: Deer Style*)

The Six Best Sex Positions Exercise

Trying out new positions may very well bring new heights of pleasure to both of you, and it's so very playful. Some positions may bring laughter into your bedroom when you find that a new position does not suit either of you—at least on the first try.

Motivational Moment

Of course everyone is different, but the benefit of finding a position that you both feel is the best for you is untold. Trying new positions is pure fun, of course, and finally finding a position that seems to be the best will be beneficial for both of you.

Note About The Six Best Sex Positions

In this chapter, you learned position after position that will enable both of you to feel G-spot stimulation, thus bringing you both more pleasure. The sexual pleasure you will get from the different positions is related to how intensely the clitoris, G-spot, or A-spot can be stimulated. This depends upon the physical shape and positions of the erogenous spots of each woman (as well as upon her ability to relax during intercourse) and the thickness and length of the man's penis, as well as the hardness of each erection. Trying will bring variety to your sex life, and you will find the position that suits you best for your pleasure.

Fill in this log to keep a record of the results of your exercises:

1. Which position did you do this week: The Surprise, The Organ Grinder, The Yab Yum, Deep Impact, Doggy Style, Deer Style?

2. What change do you want to see in yourself spiritually and sexually?

3. How do you feel about your own sexuality now that you have done these exercises?

4. On a scale of 1 to 10, with 10 the maximum, how have these exercises improved the quality of your orgasm(s)?

	1	2	3	4
Week 1				
Week 2				
Week 3				
Week 4				
Week 5				
Week 6				
Week 7				
Week 8				

CHAPTER 13

Date with Your Lover

Whether you are married or not, regular dates with your lover are a necessity to keep the fires burning. By setting aside time specifically for connecting with each other, you not only maintain your relationship but grow even closer to one another.

Make a Date

Set aside one day or night every week to spend with your lover. Fancy plans are not necessary, but the occasional surprise can certainly help heat things up in the bedroom. It is extremely important to stick to these dates as often as possible, as they are essential to your relationship.

Revisit the Old Days

Think about what you did for your spouse when you were first dating. Did you sneak little peeks when you thought he or she wasn't looking? Reach for his or her hand or arm as often as possible to show everyone around who you were with? Or perhaps you were more accommodating in making plans for your dates? Whatever it was that you used to do, try to bring those actions back, and your partner will be pleasantly surprised.

Dress to Impress

Go out and purchase a slinky little number just for an upcoming date. Shave in all the necessary places before your date, and moisturize, moisturize, moisturize! Do everything you can to not only look hot, but feel like a sexy vixen, too!

- Pluck your eyebrows.
- Use a depilatory for any facial hair.
- Add sparkle to your hairdo with some glitter.
- Paint your nails and toenails with the color your partner likes best on them.
- Layer on a sexy perfume. Too much will take his breath away in a bad way!

Variety Is the Spice of Life

If you and your partner are in a rut when it comes to dating destinations, there are plenty of options that both of you may enjoy. Dates are not limited to dinner and a movie. Consider some of the following ideas:

- Pack a picnic with your husband's favorite foods and make out in a secluded area.
- Attend tango or salsa classes. Not only will you learn a new dance, but the spicy moves required by these dances are sure to extend into your love life as well.
- Find a secluded place to park, and enjoy each other in the backseat.

- Visit a sex boutique, and ask your man if there is anything there that interests him.
- Go to an ethnic festival. Pick up some interesting clothing items and wonder about their mysterious purpose.

Home Can Be Hot Too

Don't be afraid to plan a date to stay at home. There are plenty of date ideas that will turn the heat up on your relationship in the comfort of your own home. Consider the following:

- Taste-test aphrodisiac foods such as oysters and chocolate fondue. Find out if these work for either of you.
- Take a bath together. Light candles and add bubble bath for a luxurious soak. And remember: There is no rule against sex in the bathtub!
- Give your lover a massage, complete with edible massage oil.
- Play a game of strip poker. It may seem juvenile, but it can certainly get your juices flowing!
- Model your lingerie. This is the perfect excuse to purchase the lingerie of your dreams!

Take Turns Planning Dates

Alternating the date planning allows for even more anticipation of the Big Day. By planning activities that you know will please your partner, you show that you truly do listen and that you want your partner to be happy. Note that men typically have different interests than women, so don't be afraid to play off of that.

- Plan a golf outing. It really doesn't matter if you have no golf skills; Just the thought of having such beautiful company will please any man.

- Purchase tickets to a sporting event, but don't tell him where you are going.

- Test drive some unreasonably priced cars. You'll both need to dress to the nines and act unbearably rich.

- Go to a theme park and let your spouse choose all the rides. The adrenaline rush will keep both of you hyped for hours.

- Plan a camping trip. Take care of all the packing so that all your spouse has to do is put on his baseball cap.

Anniversaries

The most special date ideas should be saved for anniversaries. This special day only comes once a year, so make it memorable.

- Recreate your first date. If you no longer live in the same area, duplicate your first date as closely as possible. The date needn't have been exceptional; the fact that it was your first date makes it inherently romantic.

- Recall your wedding meal. Complete with a small punch fountain, recreate your wedding reception meal. Don't forget to have a small decorated cake to cut together.

- Book a romantic photo shoot. Dress up in sexy clothes, and choose your spouse's most flattering clothes. Don't be afraid to show a little skin!

Caress your lover

For those of you who have been in a relationship for a while and you feel that you are getting into a routine in the bedroom, those who feel they have lost the attraction for each other, or those who are just starting a relationship and are excited about exploring slowly your partner's body. I recommend a wonderful technique called Karezza. This term is the Italian equivalent of the word "caress" and it includes a lot of cuddling, spooning, skin-on-skin contact, hugs, soft petting, and gentle intercourse.

Karezza is the orgasm of the soul. It uses to be the way to sacred sex, as well as Tantric sex to practice male orgasm control. It was reintroduced in our western world by Alice Bunker Stockham.

In our western society Karezza is not as rigorous as the Taoist philosophy repressing male orgasm and letting the female having as many orgasms as she desire since the woman is already born Goddess. Karezza is a practice that puts aside the orgasm as a goal, and introduces the goal as being the exploration itself, the peace and love, the union with your partner.

Today males and females may have orgasm. The concept is very much a free style caress, to make love slowly and gently be attentive to each others breathing and relaxing and welcoming an orgasm if any occurs, and if none occur it is also fine. Karezza is to realize that our entire creature: body, mind and soul is one and it is one great erogenous zone. During Karezza practice, you may feel at peace, happy, satisfied, in love, floating. You can practice Karezza with your partner in order to rediscover their body, release the sexual energy and let it flow through your body, unite your souls, or simply for caressing each other. It is important to avoid genital stimulation. The happiness and the feeling of peace and connection come from the release of oxytocin, also called "the cuddle hormone". This hormone is released during embraces, soft touches, gentle intercourse, all of these being included into the Karezza practice. What exactly does this practice means and how can you experience it?

- With the lights dimmed and wearing no clothes, lay facing your partner. Start caressing your partner with your palm or the tips of your fingers. You can use eye contact while touching each other, or keep your eyes closed, in order to focus on your sensations.

- In Karezza, the man should be in control and have initiative, and the woman should find herself supportive, both as energy and as practice. This does not mean that the man dominates the woman, but that the man represents the active, more strong principle (the yang), and the woman is the soft, receiving principle (the yin). This way, they complete and balance each other.

- Explore your partner's body for a period of twenty minutes to two hours.

- Caress each other from head to toe. Soft and gentle kisses, touches and intercourse are recommended in order to provide the necessary amount of time to explore each other's body patiently and quietly.

Through Karezza, your relationship becomes stronger and so does the attractiveness. By exploring each other's body, you are always surprised and excited, even if you have been married for ten or twenty years. You will observe that you are less irritable, you fight less with your partner, and you appreciate each other's company more. It is a practice for both people at the beginning of a relationship and for long-term, steady couples. As a sensuality intimacy coach I often recommend Karezza practice. One couple who's marriage was based on deep love for each other but unfortunately was completely sexless, practiced Karezza for over a period of a few weeks to two years and then returned to a very explosive sex life.

Exercise for Dating Your Lover

Plan a date for your husband to remember. Dress up in the sexiest outfit you have, and primp to the extreme. You want your husband to start salivating when he first sees you. Fight off his advances, and inform him that you have a special date planned for him.

He will be expecting to be taken to a fancy dinner, so surprise him by going to a sports bar or even a strip club, if you don't mind.

- Order food that you lick or engulf with your mouth, to get him thinking about what you can do to him.

- Give his order to the waiter for him, and order a bottle of wine or champagne. Offer a toast to the two of you.

- If you are in a strip club, surprise him with a lap dance.

- Lead your husband on to believe that this is it for the night, and that you will be going home after your special date.

- Follow up dinner with a trip to a comedy club. Try to find a relatively secluded spot where you can fondle your man without anyone noticing. When he just can't take it anymore, agree to leave, but insist on going straight home. (No getting it on in the car!)

At home, insist on giving him a back massage before anything else. Make him wait for his pleasure, and he will be practically ready to explode! Have on hand some new sex toys or lotions, and you will both remember this date night for a long time!

Motivational Moment

Regardless of your budget, the most important thing when planning a date night is to make it a priority. There are plenty of low-cost or even no-cost ideas that are sure to improve your love life. Try one of these for your next date, and you just may be surprised at the results!

If your love life has become predictable, if you remember that you used to be so much in love and so orgasmic, but these days you rarely (or never) reach orgasm, spicing things up outside the bedroom can have incredible benefits for your sex life. By increasing your intimacy in general, you will feel more in tune with your partner, increasing your ability to reach orgasm.

Note About Dates with Your Lover

Is your relationship in a rut? This chapter gave you plenty of unique ideas for some hot, sexy dates to get both you and your partner randy. By taking the time to plan for a memorable night, you can practically insure that both of you will be beyond ready for an orgasm when the time comes.

Fill in this log to keep a record of the results of your exercises.

1. Which of these date exercises did you do this week: Make a Date? Dress to Impress? Pack a picnic? Attend tango or salsa classes? Find a secluded place? Visit a sex boutique? Go to an ethnic festival? Taste-test aphrodisiac foods? Take a bath together? Give your lover a massage? Play a game of strip poker? Model your lingerie? Plan a golf outing? Purchase tickets to a sporting event? Plan a camping trip? Recreate your first date? Book a romantic photo shoot? Did you practice the Karezza technique?

2. What change do you want to see in yourself spiritually and sexually?

3. How do you feel about your own sexuality now you have done these exercises?

4. On a scale of 1 to 10, with 10 the maximum, how have these exercises improved the quality of your orgasm(s)?

	1	2	3	4
Week 1				
Week 2				
Week 3				
Week 4				
Week 5				
Week 6				
Week 7				
Week 8				

CHAPTER 14

Tantra Quickies

If you are part of the 80 percent of women in this world who have both a job and a family, you know that this era of speed in which we currently live sometimes makes it impossible to breathe properly, let alone have time for exploring the sensual world of Tantra. "Tantra quickies" might seem like an oxymoron, because when it comes to Tantra, you think about making love with your partner for hours and enjoying each other's company for an entire night. As you may have found out already, Tantra is only partly about sexuality; the rest is about spirituality and becoming one with your partner. This is why Tantra quickies will show you how to bring spirituality and the intensity of Tantric lovemaking into your life and allow you to indulge in sexual nirvana.

If you are wondering what, exactly, a Tantra quickie is, here are some of the answers that several women gave me:

- A short exercise to improve your sensuality.

- A moment for you and your partner to remember your love.

- A moment of emotional and sexual foreplay.

- A simple technique to keep the love spark alive for you as a couple.

Although from time to time it would be best to clear your agenda and spend some time with scented candles, massage oils, and a patient partner, the rest of the time you can use Tantra quickies to keep your emotional and sexual connection between yourself and your partner. The best part is that each of the exercises in the short list below only takes ten minutes! Use your imagination and create other exercises that boost both your sexuality and your intimacy; anything that makes you feel good about yourself and your relationship will do. The only rule is to keep it under ten minutes.

1. Bring your partner breakfast in bed, and wake him or her with lots of kisses all over his body.

2. While at work, send your partner a text message or email with a short but very personal description of a fantasy you would like to try when she gets home. Talk about what you did to her the last time you were together. Tell her how hard you are for her. Talk about velvet tongue on her clit. I don't know one woman who is not turn on by an erotic text or message. She will leave her job earlier only to be pleasured by expert fingers, tongue and penis.

3. Delight your partner with ten minutes of oral sex. Although this may seem too short, the purpose is not orgasm but pleasure and surprise—and anticipation!

4. Stare into each other's eyes for ten minutes, without saying a word. Try expressing your love and desire through your eyes.

5. Make love in the morning. After brief foreplay, choose a position that allows you to gaze into each other's eyes. Again, the purpose (especially for men) is not the climax but your connection and intimacy.

You and your partner should introduce these Tantra quickies in your life together, and practice them on a daily basis. Do not be afraid to experiment and add other techniques that will improve your sexual and emotional connection. These may not seem like big changes because they only take ten minutes a day, but if you try them for a couple of weeks, you will see their miraculous advantages:

- Your sexual energy will be awakened and increased.

- When making love, you will get aroused more easily than before.

- Men will improve their control over their ejaculations, and learn to recirculate their sexual energy rather than ejaculate fast.

- Your communication and intimacy levels will be highly improved.

- You will start observing that you have more time for yourself and for yourselves as a couple.

Not only do these Tantra quickies improve your relationship, they also boost your self-confidence, your self-image, and your level of endorphins, which will make you happy overall.

Exercise for Tantra Quickies

Take the first step, and include in your daily program at least one Tantra quickie of your choice. Practice it every day for a week and see what happens with yourself and your relationship. When the week is over, try two Tantra quickies daily from the list above or those invented by you and your partner. Look at the quickies not as chores, but as a fun way to keep the flame of your love alive. With time, include another quickie and then another one, and soon you will have a smile upon your face for the entire day.

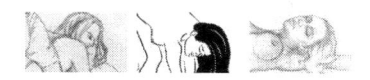

Motivational Moment

Even if you have a busy job or you have to take care of the house and children, the lack of time is not an excuse any more for not exploring the magic of Tantra. You can improve your sexual and emotional life right now. Ten minutes a day is all you need to begin to see the benefits of Tantra quickies. Your relationship will improve, your self-esteem will rise, and your sensuality will blossom.

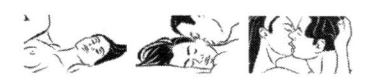

Note About Tantra Quickies

This chapter is for all the women who feel they say the phrase, "I'm too busy!" far too often. You've learned how to include in your life as part of a couple some short, simple, easy-to-follow Tantra practices that will boost your relationship both emotionally and sexually.

Fill in this log to keep a record of the results of your exercises:

1. Which of these Tantra quickies did you do this week: Bring your partner breakfast in bed? Send your partner a text message with a short description of a fantasy you would like to try when he gets home? Ten minutes of oral sex? Make love in the morning?

2. What change do you want to see in yourself spiritually and sexually?

3. How do you feel about your own sexuality now that you have done these exercises?

4. On a scale of 1 to 10, with 10 the maximum, how have these exercises improved the quality of your orgasm(s)?

	1	2	3	4
Week 1				
Week 2				
Week 3				
Week 4				
Week 5				
Week 6				
Week 7				
Week 8				

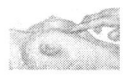

CHAPTER 15

Fetishism, Fantasies and Role Playing in the Tantric World

I was on my way to a little Motel 6 out in Orange County. The woman who had called me described herself as a widow who, at fifty-three, was giving up. The business she was running was close to shutting its doors, and sexually she felt trapped.

I arrived at the motel to find a room key waiting for me. I rode the elevator, carefully planning my moves like a chess master. I wanted to have every touch and approach planned out in my head, so that I could deliver a first-class, truly relaxing experience to my client.

I entered the room and was hit by how dark it was. The heavy curtains were drawn, and the only light came from the low-voltage reading lamps on either side of the bed.

"Hi, Jean-Claude," Cinnamon said to me, as I walked over to the bed. "You said it was time to pamper myself, so I thought, Why not go the whole way and really blow my own mind?'." Cinnamon smiled as she spoke, and in the dull light I thought that maybe she had even winked. "I told I would have a little surprise for you," she smiled. On the bed she *had laid out all the gear for a perfect BDSM evening: ropes, handcuffs, gags and muzzles, a blindfold, a hood, and whips.*

"I trust you are going to do a good job on me," Cinnamon continued. "It is the only way that my mind can be stimulated these days."

The secret world of fetishism and bondage is larger than we imagine. I was aware that a person who enjoys bondage walks a very fine line between pain, excitement, danger, and trust. It is in that very narrow zone that she will ultimately find her pleasure.

I had been in this situation before. I read Cinnamon's mind in the shyness of her eyes, and I knew what she secretly wanted. She would try her best to show me that she was stronger than me, and I was to let her get her way—for a while—to please her. She will smile thinking I found "my bitch".

At some point, I would have to show her that I would let her get away with nothing. Then she would feel trapped, hopeless, useless, degraded with a complete sense of failure. Her mind would let her body go, accepting and recognizing that I am her ultimate master. She will be on her knees, accepting she met her ultimate power. She will know that I will always be more powerful than her. At that point only she will begin to enjoy the most, erotic, pleasurable and orgasmic night she had had for a long time. . . .

Despite suppression by today's society, fetishism is generally not a harmful fixation. An individual can have a fetish for almost anything, from feet or shoes to leather or lace. In addition, the intensity of a fetish varies from person to person, making generalization difficult. But playing along with a fetish can greatly enhance a woman's ability to have more frequent and more intense orgasms. Often a fetishism take its roots in our childhood, like the first time the child suck the heel of her mother shoes, or was spanked by her father,

By allowing your mind to embrace the sensuality of different fetishistic acts and materials, you open the door to a literally mind-blowing orgasm. Identifying what turns you on mentally and then using it physically, allow you to experience an orgasm in more than one sphere of your being, amplifying the sensations tenfold.

Different Types of Fetishes

Hair Fetish: Cindy emailed me, "*Dear Jean-Claude, My most erogenous zone, besides my mind, would be my nipples, my feet, my clit, and believe it or not, having my hair on my head stroked/pulled/brushed. When I was a little girl, I remember someone sitting behind me in class, I think I was in 3rd grade, and he/she (don't remember who) was playing with my hair. I felt a little turned on, and didn't know what was happening, but this has been a feeling that I have never forgotten. It's not hard, not pulling hard, and not timidly gentle, it's just having my hair pulled into a pony tail, and caressed. I always have wanted to share this with my lover, but with you it is different.*"

Many men have hair fetishes and are easily turned on just by the sight of long, silky tresses. If you don't have extremely long hair, you can still utilize your hair to amplify your sex life. Just tousling your hair to give yourself that post coital look can turn both you and your partner on. During foreplay, place your man's hands in your hair and rub them around. Encouraging him to pull your hair a bit can be a major turn-on. Tickle your partner's sensitive areas with your hair, and you will both be ready to go, quickly!

Silk Fetish: A silk fetish can be pleasurable for both partners. Consider dressing up in a sexy silk lingerie number for a simple fix, or invest in a quality silk scarf in a passionate color such as red. Greet your partner with this around your neck, and you will instantly have his attention.

The material will feel amazing on your soft, silky skin, as well as on a man's rougher skin. Feel free to get playful, and do a little dance for your man, ending by rubbing the scarf between your legs to get both of you riled up for a spicy night.

Foot Fetish: Every man loves soft, well-cared-for feet on a woman. Keep your toenails painted and prepped for an unexpected tryst. Besides attracting your partner, every woman feels sexier with gorgeous feet. Use your feet to your benefit when making love. After all, women's toes are incredibly flexible and with some practice, you will find that you can even get your partner off with some fancy footwork against his privates. Running your foot against the hairy legs of your man not only can turn him on, but can make you feel even more like the sex Goddess you are.

Public Sex: Few couples do not get turned on by the idea of getting caught having sex in public. Although many couples are afraid of the risks, there are a number of ways to accommodate this taste with minimal risk that will still keep the adrenaline flowing. For example, many hotels have a whirlpool in addition to their swimming pool. Some place these are in a relatively secluded area, making sex in a hot tub a very real (and hot) option on less popular travel days, such as midday on a weekday. Another great idea is to find an unmonitored dressing room and enjoy a secret quickie.

Mirrors: Some people simply can't have an orgasm without seeing themselves in a mirror. By positioning a mirror next to or above the bed, anyone can take advantage of this fetish. Being able to see yourself enjoying sex can be an immense turn-on, and you can switch positions with your partner throughout lovemaking to give both of you a chance to enjoy the view.

Blindfolds and Handcuffs: Handcuffs and blindfolds are popular tools to use in the bedroom. To indulge in this fetish, you can simply use a scarf or piece of fabric as a blindfold, and purchase an inexpensive pair of handcuffs. Be sure to use handcuffs that do not require a key for release, or you may be faced with some interesting explanations for the local locksmith! Use both of these items on your partner and do whatever you want to him. Many women find this a turn-on, squirting chocolate syrup all over their partner and slowly choosing where to lick it off. Your partner's anticipation will cause him to strain at the handcuffs, and he'll find it so pleasurable that he'll be sure to reciprocate.

Bondage: Bondage is becoming increasingly accepted as an addition to anyone's sex life. Ranging from such mild forms as simply tying a partner's ankles together to extreme forms such as placing a partner in a body bag, most couples choose to introduce the simplest forms of this fetish into their sex life initially. Ask your partner to tie your wrists above your head while he licks whipped topping from all of your favorite places, and you will quickly learn how pleasurable bondage can be.

Spanking: Few men will shoot down a woman who requests to be punished by a good spanking, but first you might want to show him how it's done. Spanking is often used in role-playing such as "Principal and Student," or similar fantasies. (*see drawing: Spanking is often used in role-playing such as "Principal and Student," or similar fantasies*) A good introduction of this into foreplay would be to begin with a bit of a warm-up, with light spanking of the cheeks or rubbing. For a different feeling, you can place some petroleum jelly or even syrup on the cheeks. Dramatic pauses increase your partner's expectation, along with increasing intensity. Be sure to keep it relatively mild though, especially in the beginning, as too much pain can be a complete turn-off. Once you have taught your partner a lesson, switch positions, being sure to give him verbal feedback as to how you like it. The first orgasm of the girl may have been when her father spank her. This could be due to the stimulation of her clitoris against the legs of her father. (*see drawing: Spanking*)

High Heels: High heel fetishes are common in both men and women. High heels by their very nature make a woman's legs look like they go on forever, and the wearer feels incredibly sexy. Try wearing the highest heels you can, and if you can find some that have satin laces that crisscross up your legs, you will drive your man wild with desire. Pair these with the shortest miniskirt you can find, without underwear. Sex with high heels on is incredibly hot, and if you choose to be on top in this tryst, you can easily keep your miniskirt on and feel even naughtier. If you or your partner enjoy a little pain during sex, heels can be used anywhere on the body for some painful pleasure.

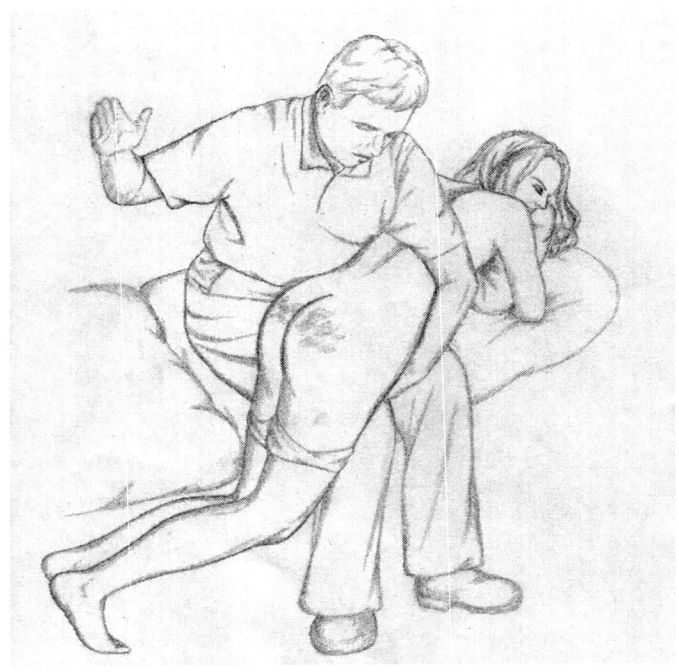

Spanking is often used in role-playing such as "Principal and Student," or similar fantasies

Sex during Pregnancy and Lactation: During pregnancy, if your doctor does not recommend otherwise, you are perfectly able to have sex until the last day of pregnancy. The libido fluctuates during pregnancy, but most women experience a growth in their sexual appetite during the second trimester, after the morning sickness is gone. You may also feel more relaxed and willing to experiment with your partner. Also, helping your mate by bringing her to orgasm during labor (not through penetration, but with your mouth or hand) will attenuate pain and release endorphins, which have a calming effect. If your belly is getting bigger, there is no need to feel frustrated. Here are some positions and sexual practices that will satisfy your appetite during those nine long months:

- Doggy style: you on your knees and hands, with your partner penetrating you from behind. This is a great position to try, as your belly is protected, and the deep penetration will stimulate your G-spot.

- Cunnilingus: Most women become more sensitive during their pregnancy, and this is why you will most likely enjoy cunnilingus even more than before.

- Tantric massage: Using only soft touches, your partner can caress your body from head to toe, using the techniques described in Chapter 3.

After the birth, if you are into it, you can try lactation (breastfeeding from your partner). Most women find the act of having their nipples sucked while lactating highly arousing and erotic. To help the milk come out, take the breast into your hands, and gently squeeze it toward your mouth while sucking on the nipple. Be gentle at first, and then add more suction. Your partner might love it. If you both like it, the lactation period can be prolonged by massaging the breast and suckling.

Trying out some of the ideas based on fetishes can increase sexual pleasure for both you and your partner. Besides just spicing up your sex life, exploring new areas of your sexuality brings you and your partner closer as a couple, allowing for more meaningful and intense orgasms.

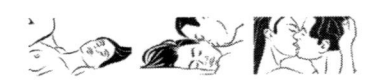

Fetishism Exercise

If you and your partner have not experimented much in the bedroom so far, start with one of the tamer ideas, such as wearing sky-high heels and keeping them on during sex, or bringing a silk scarf to bed. These ideas are so subdued that you may wish to surprise your partner, especially if he loves your high-heeled shoes? For some of the more extreme fetishes such as bondage and handcuffs, be sure to talk with your partner before trying them, or you could face a night of arguing rather than one of enjoyment. Be aware that the best part of sex, in general, is about discovering what brings pleasure to each other. Talking and coaching men and women, addressing their separate issues, both tell me, "*She (or he) was so boring in bed, and there was no imagination at all. My new lover (or my mistress) knows exactly how to bring me pleasure.*"

Unfortunately trust has nothing to do with the time spent together, but a sense of chemistry that is either there or not from the beginning. Chemistry is one of the reasons couples divorce after many years in a relationship, and this is often a great surprise for one of the partners. Often I hear, "*I trusted him (or her) so much,*" but in the end, most people want to be with the one he or she has the best sex with. The bottom line for both men and women is that they should learn through Tantra how to keep their mates. Become irresistible and a great lover, and then you will never have to wonder or feel insecure. You will know that you have everything you need to keep the man or woman you love around.

Motivational Moment

Whether you are a man or a woman, try one of the fetish ideas above tonight and surprise your partner with a new sexual experience. Many of these ideas are inexpensive and require minimal preparation, making them easy to implement and ideal for helping to take your orgasm to the next level.

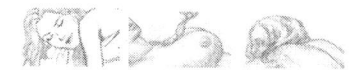

Note About Fetishism

If you are looking to spice up your sex life and enjoy orgasms in an entirely different way, consider trying some fetish ideas. By implementing ideas that stimulate both your mind and your body, your sexual experience can be amplified to an unbelievable extent.

Fill in this log to keep a record of the results of your exercises:

1. Which fetish exercise did you do this week: Hair Fetish? Silk Fetish? Public Sex? Mirrors? Blindfolds and Handcuffs? Bondage? Spanking? High Heels? Or maybe something else?

2. What change do you want to see in yourself spiritually and sexually?

3. How do you feel about your own sexuality now you have done these exercises?

4. On a scale of 1 to 10, with 10 the maximum, how have these exercises improved the quality of your orgasm(s)?

	1	2	3	4
Week 1				
Week 2				
Week 3				
Week 4				
Week 5				
Week 6				
Week 7				
Week 8				

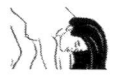

CHAPTER 16

Goodbye and Good Morning

The Goodbye Part

One of human beings' defining characteristics is emotion, which runs the gamut from great joy to overwhelming sadness. The reasons for sadness can be various: a breakup, the death of a lover, or any other hurtful emotional experience. Experiences that evoke feelings of sadness also are often associated with anger, distress, regret, or remorse. Unfortunately, Western-style education, which is mainly based on rationalism and issues from Descartes and later Cartesian philosophy, doesn't leave much space within which to become aware of our spirituality and emotions. Therefore most of us are not well prepared to experience a state of overwhelming sorrow.

We so often feel self-conscious and shy about our emotional distress; we even take it as a sign of fragility and failure, even though we know on a rational level that strong emotions such as sadness are part of our existence. The best medicine would be to open the heart's door to someone who cares. We should let go loudly until we feel the pain has begun to heal and realize that emotion is not a duality with life, but a part of the process of our existence; indeed, the "negative" emotions we try to avoid even acknowledging, are essential if we are to later feel joy and happiness.

After you have taken some time to integrate the loss of your lover—or indeed, of any loss, whatever its nature may be—you may try to rediscover your inner sensuality, your inner Goddess. Start practicing Tantric breathing and meditation, as well as self-exploration and self-pleasuring. All of these will help you when you are ready to open your heart to a new lover.

Here are a few things that you can do after a breakup in order to ease the pain and help you integrate your separation:

- Make a list of all the beautiful things in your relationship, as well as all of the things that put the two of you on different pages in life. Make another list of all the things that you have learned from that relationship. From a partner who was busy and always on the road, you could, for example, learn to appreciate the moments you will have with your new partner.

- Look at the situation as a challenge. Each experience teaches us something new that will help us evolve spiritually and emotionally. Try to find the lesson hidden in your loss.

- Enumerate your needs and your ex-partner's needs, and try to understand why you could not fulfill these needs for each other. Use this knowledge to choose a new partner whose needs are similar to yours.

- Look toward your future. It is difficult to step forward and see what is ahead of you if your eyes are constantly looking back.

- Here are a few steps to guide you in the process of mourning:

- Cry. Do not be afraid to show your suffering; this does not make you weak but strong. Tears are a wonderful emotional cleanser, and it is okay to let them flow.

- Write a letter to your partner. Write him everything you feel, all of your thoughts and pain. Just let yourself put everything on that piece of paper, until you feel you have nothing more to say. Then send it into the universe in a symbolic way: Make a paper boat out of it and put it in the river, burn it, bury it—whatever comes naturally to you. This is not a letter for the soul of your partner, but a letter for your own soul.

- When you no longer feel angry and hurt, but you simply miss him, have a gathering with your closest friends to look at family pictures and share happy memories of him in different stages of life. Being with people who also miss him will soothe your longing and celebrate his life.

The death of a very close loved one may result in loss of sexuality and depression for some time. However, our minds generally are strong and well balanced enough to recover reasonably rapidly. However, it may happen that a year has passed after your loss, and you still find yourself often feeling vulnerable, depressed, or emotionally and sexually unavailable for a new relationship. If this is the case, you may need professional advice; becoming locked in this pattern could become dangerous for the healthy functioning of your mind and body. Do not hesitate to talk to your family doctor, who will advise you on the best way forward for your recovery.

Living Your Good Morning!

Depending on your past and traumatic experiences, sometimes even a new relationship is not easy .Once a woman feels she has failed one too many times to find the right man, she becomes more cautious and less trustful of the male gender and also less confident in herself. The sense of joy in a new relationship also could be associated with a feeling of fear. The following email that I received could describe the way that many women may experience their emotional life.

"Thank you for your enlightening emails. You have opened so much repressed energy just by explaining about feminine sexuality, and by doing so have caused feelings of vulnerability to surface."

"I was very sexually active as a teenager following my rape. I was molested as a young girl and raped several times over the years, from date rape, to stranger rape at gunpoint, and even a gang rape. I married and was sexually unhappy. After my husband was murdered, I had affairs in which sex was the only exercise I did regularly. In writing this, I realize that I have never had a man really make love to me, joining together sexually as a spiritual union of love. It was love in the moment; I know you understand exactly what I mean."

"Sex, for me, was at times an empowering act to make a man weak. I tried to use him instead of letting him use me. Don't get me wrong—I've been in a few committed relationships, but sex together was never about pleasuring me; it was about him. I had both male and female partners, as well as threesomes, and I even sold my body in prostitution."

"I have found, following an early menopause, that I am not as aroused as I used to be. As I sit here and write to you, the sadness I feel makes me cry. This always happens when I open myself up. My environment is a mess, but my spirit is undaunted. I find I am not concerned by appearances, or by what a person does or with who."

"Three months ago, for the first time in my life, I met a beautiful man who really loves me for who I am. I am also really in love for the first time in my life. I know he is ready to propose that I marry him, but frankly, I am panicking. I truly believe that, with your help, I could handle the situation with calm without making the same mistakes all over again. I need your coaching and advices urgently."

"Waiting to hear from you,

"Linda."

When you meet the person that both your heart and body crave, a journey full of wonder and beauty lies ahead—that is, if you make it wondrous and beautiful. A strong emotional and sexual connection builds up from the first date, so here are a few tips to follow to make sure your intimacy levels will be running high pretty soon:

- Pick a song that you feel speaks about your relationship and make it "our song," Every time you hear it, dance together, no matter where you find yourselves at that moment.

- Hold hands when going out. Even if you have an open or nonconformist relationship, this habit will help you by raising your endorphin levels and consolidating your intimacy.

- Develop a hobby together. Find some common interest, and share it, whether it is a sport, travelling, or clubbing.

- Compliment each other at least once a day. You can praise the choice of movie rentals or the way you make each other feel in bed, but just do it. Compliments boost self-esteem and self-worth and give you the feeling that you can tell each other everything.

- When in a new relationship, you will experience the thrill of your first sexual experience together—with the advantage of knowing what you are doing this time. If you want to make sure that you and your partner will have a fulfilling sexual life, here are some tips to follow from the very first night you have sex:

For a woman

- Explore your partner every time with tenderness and curiosity, as though you are trying to imprint the shape of his body in the tips of your fingers. Create a mental map of his body, and discover his erogenous areas.

- Take time to experiment together, and try different positions and touches in order to get to know each other's sexual preferences and improve your experience. Leave inhibitions aside.

- Communication is the key, both in nonsexual relationships and in sexual ones. Let your partner know what you need, either with words or by showing him directly. He will appreciate the tips and feel more sexually secure in your relationship.

- Before, you enter in the bedroom tell him to enjoy your body in no rush, he needs to explore your sensuality from head to toes. But most importantly tell him you come first. Otherwise, no second chance.

For a man

- As a man you are used to go from point A to point B and you are born to resolve problems. A woman wants to be listened to, and a man should learn to listen to his woman. Listen, do not offer her your solution. She will find her own solution, which often will be completely opposite to a man's logic. She will say thank you for listening.

- Be attentive when you look at her, don't look all over the place when you have a coffee or dinner date with your future Goddess. Look at her in her eyes, look at her face and be attentive at her words. Take mental notes of what she likes and dislikes, and use it for your next date. Prepare strawberry, mango if it's a favorite fruits or learn how to make a real mojito if she told you she loved that drink in summer time with fresh mint leaves. I guarantee she will start to speak to you in Spanish in no time. Bust most of all, she will know that when you will make love you will be focus totally on her pleasure.

- Let her have her orgasm before yours. Be aware that she always comes first. Together, it's even better of course.

- Be a "bad boy" in the bedroom, slowly open her to talk dirty to you, she will love it. What is in the bedroom stay in the bedroom. But be courteous outside of the bedroom. Please and thank you are very short words which will show that you are educated but mostly will create a positive connection and she will want to see you again.

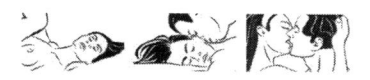

Exercises for Goodbye and Good Morning

Put the things that remind you of your lost love in a box: pictures, clothes, the tickets from your first movie date, and so on. If you have no real objects, use a symbolic one such as a broken heart card. Tape the box shut, and write on it, "Beautiful memories." Then deposit the box in the attic or in a place where you do not go often. Memories from a relationship are a wonderful gift, and we should treasure them, but it can be difficult to find room for a new partner in a house or soul full of old memories.

Think of sexual experience as sampling a fine food: You should have all of your five senses involved. Try using all of them during your next sexual experience. Watch your partner's body and gestures, ask him to whisper words in your ear, sniff his scent, lick his skin to feel his taste, touch him using not only your hands but your whole body, because your skin is your largest receptive organ. Your brain will be flooded with these opulent stimuli, and you will experience a state of bliss.

Motivational Moment

A great part of life is to accept the things that we cannot change, and a lost love can be one of those things. If grieving for a lost love is consuming your energy—the energy that should feed your emotional and sexual self—now you can stop grieving and move on to rediscover your femininity and sensuality. Encountering and welcoming a new lover is part of the wonder that life can offer to us. Don't miss the enjoyment of a new relationship and build a beautiful connection. Look for a rainbow in your heart. You know you deserve it.

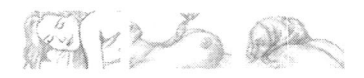

Note About "Goodbye and Good Morning"

If you have ever been through a breakup, lost a loved partner, and been hurt, this chapter is for you. Here you have found out how to let go of your unrequited love, how to accept that your partner does not love you anymore, or how to live on and start again after your partner has passed away. Once you put your life together and find a new love, the tips offered here will help you with building your intimacy with your partner and improve your emotional and sexual connection.

Fill in this log to keep a record of the results of your exercises:

1. Which Goodbye and Good Morning exercises did you do this week: Make a list of all the beautiful things in your relationship? Look at the situation as a challenge? Look toward your future? Cry? Show your suffering? Write a letter for your partner? Pick a song that speaks to your new relationship? Hold hands when going out? Develop a hobby together? Compliment each other at least once a day? Explore your partner every time with tenderness and curiosity? Take time to experiment together? Or maybe something else?

2. What change do you want to see in yourself spiritually and sexually?

3. How do you feel about your own sexuality now you have done these exercises?

4. On a scale of 1 to 10, with 10 the maximum, how have these exercises improved the quality of your orgasm(s)?

	1	2	3	4
Week 1				
Week 2				
Week 3				
Week 4				
Week 5				
Week 6				
Week 7				
Week 8				

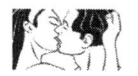

CONCLUSION

One day a lady wrote to me, saying, "*Sex is sex, but after sex there is nothing left. Maybe Tantra is what I need to go deeper into myself and feel a sexual union with my partner.*"

You are now aware that there is no special technique in Tantra, but that you can go as deep as the freedom of your mind will allow you to go. In fact, there is no limit until you touch the real core of your sexuality, because we are all Tantric in ourselves. The pavement of our daily lives has bruised and built our egos, and we became what we became. Tantra is to open your heart and your soul and become a part of your partner, and for him or her to become a part of you.

The evolution of our humanity started from our consciousness. For us to be able to evolve as better humans, we have to direct ourselves to a higher level of consciousness. Tantra is a step on the way to a higher consciousness.

Sometime, our sexual problems with a partner stem from relying upon nonverbal communication and from our egos. For example, you may feel like bragging to your partner that you now know something about Tantra that he doesn't. Resist that impulse coming from your ego; it will be much nicer and further the cause of intimacy to simply share something you feel, which will be a pleasure for both of you.

Start to communicate with your partner by noticing things and asking questions, but go slowly: We are very fragile, and we do not open so easily. Show your partner that his or her pleasure is your pleasure as well. Then you will be able to find a solution to your many sexual questions that you believe may be problems. Those supposed problems usually are only a misunderstanding with your partner. If you love him, do not stop communicating with him. This will be your first step toward your ecstatic journey in Tantra.

Despite all that you have learned in this book, do not forget that your brain remains your best sex organ. Your brain, however, can either limit your sexuality or open you up to a completely different dimension. My intention has been to make you realize that your entire body, from the top of your head down to your toes, is just a great pleasure zone, and that opportunities to pleasure your partner abound.

Each person has his or her own very particular spot that has not yet been found. I am sure, now that you have finished reading this guide, that you have been practicing and have discovered some spots that I don't know about—and these may be particular only to yourself. You have shown your partner that your neck, your ears, your lips, your scalp, your hands, your breasts, and all the rest of your parts are an unlimited source of pleasure. You have realized that all of these zones need special attention (such as kissing, nuzzling, sucking, and licking, as well as nibbling and massaging!) and should not be neglected. It is a beautiful game to show your special spots to your lover and allow the thrill of discovery to drive both of you wild. The discovery of one spot leads to another discovery and to yet another.

By allowing your body to be discovered by a partner without restraint and by practicing without measure, you will soon become a fully passionate, multiple orgasmic woman who is sensual, warm, and sexy—in soul and body. Enjoying fully all the great and multiple joys that sensuality and sexuality have to offer you requires only a few passionate nights to bring pleasure back into your sexual life. A woman who gets so much pleasure from her partner won't hesitate to pleasure and recompose him much more over all his anticipation. Men should not be concerned about the reciprocity and would be surprised what a woman can do to pleasure her God.

My last words to all of the people who are looking to be loved by a male or woman partner are: When you are spending that special moment with him or her give him or her all of your attention, and most of all one of the ways to make your man feel secure is by showing him that he is the reason for your happiness. A woman wants to be adored, worship, craved sexually but most of all to be heard. Show her that you are listening, she is your Goddess. Then you will win not only her body, but most important of all, her whole heart and soul.

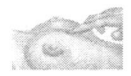

GLOSSARY

Amrita: Tantric appellation for female ejaculate.

A-spot: The anterior fornix erogenous zone (AFE zone) is an area found deep inside a woman's vagina that yields instant lubrication as well as a very long-lasting, absolutely forceful ecstasy

AFE: See A-spot.

Art therapy: A form of psychological therapy that uses different forms of art to help the client express fears and thoughts, particularly related to trauma, and then helps the client to understand and integrate the events, giving them new meaning.

Bartholin's glands: Located on either side of the lower area of the vaginal opening, these serve to secrete minor lubrication of the outer portions of the vagina to facilitate entry.

Cervix: The lowest portion of and entrance to the uterus, which is surrounded by the A-spot on the vaginal wall.

Consciousness: Awareness or openness.

Consecutive orgasms: Multiple orgasms that come one after the other, when a woman re-enters the curve of excitation through the reintroduction of stimulation after an orgasm. They require small breaks between.

Dr. Chua Chee Ann: Malaysian sex scientist who made the important discovery of the A-spot.

Energy blocks: Energy diverters that prevent thoughts and emotions from moving in a specific direction or pattern.

Endorphin: A neurotransmitter produced by the pituitary gland during exercise, excitement, pain, consumption of spicy food, love, and orgasm. It attenuates pain and produces a feeling of well-being

Fellatio: Oral sex on the lingam.

Foreskin: The prepuce that covers the tip of an uncircumcised lingam.

Glycerin-based lubes: Sugar-based lubricants that should be avoided if you are prone to yeast infections.

Goddess: According to Tantric philosophy, every woman has an inner Goddess, which contains her femininity, sensuality, and grace. (Each man also has an inner God, which contains his virility and strength.) When awakened, your inner Goddess gives you a special glow, and every gesture you make bears her mark of beauty and sensuality.

Humming: Not just for making music, humming may be used to heighten pleasure during oral sex for either a male or female.

Immunoglobulin: Immune-system antibody.

Irrumatio: A variation of fellatio in which the giver is passive and the receiver is in total control.

Kegel exercises: For men and women, these exercises involve contracting the pelvic-floor muscles to strengthen them. Strong pelvic muscles or PC muscles greatly enhance sexual pleasure and ensure the ability to control the flow of the urine with age.

Kundalini: This word comes from Sanskrit and means "coiled serpent." Kundalini is the energy that "sleeps" at the root of the spine; when awoken, it travels up the spine, opening all chakras in its way. When kundalini is aroused, a woman feels a burst of energy in her life, and her life becomes better on every level.

Lingam: Male creative energy symbolized by the male phallus.

Meatus: The opening of the urethra through which urine and ejaculate (semen) pass.

Mourning period: A time of grief over the death of someone. Mourning, in most cultures, calls for different social and religious behaviors, but its universal purpose is for the person who has lost someone to take time to pay respect to the loved one and integrate the loss.

PC (Pubococcygeus): Muscles that run from the pubic bone to the tailbone and control urine flow as well as orgasmic contractions.

Plateau: Occurs at two stages in a woman's sexual excitation curve: once before orgasm, when energy accumulates from arousal, and again after orgasm, when the body is still aroused but is preparing to return to a nonsexual state;

Point of no return: A phase in the woman's sexual excitation curve when the body's reflexive actions take over, and the woman starts to shiver, stretch her body, twitch, and so on. After this point comes orgasm.

Progressive orgasms: Multiple orgasms that come one after the other without any interruption of stimulation and with no breaks.

Psychological effect: Female ejaculation may cause a feeling of vulnerability or of calming and relaxation.

Quickie: A brief or spontaneous sexual activity that may include (but is not limited to) intercourse or oral or manual stimulation.

Reflex therapy: Also called reflexology. An Asian therapy based on massaging certain reflex points on hands and feet. Each reflex point corresponds to an internal organ; by massaging each point in a certain way, energy is released and any illness (or trauma) contained by the organs is healed.

Sanskrit: Ancient Indo-Aryan language.

Scrotum: The pouch or sac that contains the testes in males, found behind the lingam.

Sexual: Everything that has a link to or is related to sex.

Sexual consciousness: Perceived control of sexual excitation.

Sexually unavailable: Not sexually approachable by a partner. Someone who, at some moment in her or his life, does not send sexual signals to a possible partner.

Silicone-based lubes: Should not be used with silicone toys as the combination causes silicone items to break down. Cleanup is difficult, and most taste dreadful.

Solar plexus: Also called the "celiac plexus." This is the region of the abdomen where the ribs unite. The name is taken after a complex network of nerves that can be found above the stomach.

Svadhistana: The second of the seven main chakras. Svadhistana is located above the genitalia and is responsible for sexuality, sensuality, emotional fulfillment, and happy relationships.

Tantra: Asian body of belief that offers liberation from ignorance.

Trauma: Any kind of unpleasant event that leaves a deep mark in the mind. This could be the loss of someone close, a rape, domestic violence, abusive parents, emotionally abusive partners, being abandoned, and so on.

Uncircumcised: A totally uncut male who still retains the prepuce, or foreskin, of his lingam.

Urea: A chemical compound in urine.

Yoni: In Sanskrit, a woman's sexual parts.

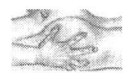

QUESTIONNAIRE

For Women Only

Be a part of history by participating in this most comprehensive sexuality questionnaire of modern times. Be honest while answering these questions. Please be over eighteen years old. You will receive by email within 24 hours your full sexual profile. It is important to understand that this questionnaire is for you to enjoy, have fun, and understand where you are with your sexuality. Many women learn a lot about themselves just by filling in the questionnaire.

http://www.mysecretquiz.com/

Did you know?

This analysis profiles the sexual habits of American women. Information has been classified according to the age, height, weight, education, occupation, marital status, and the different intimate habits of the women who answered the questionnaire. The survey reveals much about sex in our society. This report is an easy-to-understand overview of the sexual satisfaction and dissatisfaction of American women.

See the results of my analysis: http://www.mysecretquiz.com/

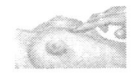

ABOUT THE AUTHOR

Jean-Claude Carvill was born in Lyon, France. He is a Beverly Hills Sensuality Intimacy Coach with over 20 years of professional experience. He is also a dedicated tantra masseur, and, since 1980, when he gave his first tantra massage, he managed to help hundreds of women to get in touch with their sexuality and become more aware of their bodies. Coming from France, Jean-Claude grew up in a more liberal and free-spirited society and had the chance to understand the importance of one's sensuality in one's life. Wanting to help women experience a fulfilled intimate life, he has traveled through Middle East, India, Southeast Asia and Australia, in order to learn the secret techniques of tantric massage. His activity grew through word-of-mouth- marketing and found its main life within circles of women with women who have a genuine desire for the growth and discovery of their sexual fulfillment. His goal is to help them with their journey to better sex, better lives and enhanced self-esteem. As an intimacy coach, Jean-Claude Carvill gives seminars on the awareness of female sexuality, but also coaches individualwomen that find themselves in a difficult spot in their relationships. Most often, women that come to Jean-Claude Carvill for sensuality coaching find it difficult to reach orgasm during intercourse, feel that they can't open themselves intimately towards their partners or they are already extremely orgasmic but wish to know if there is something more than they are already know. Through moral support and tantric techniques, Jean-Claude Carvill helps these women overcome their fears, become more aware of their bodies and their needs and have a more satisfying relationship with their partners. Those days his main activity is to work on his two books: Confessions of a Hollywood Tantra Masseur: The Untold Secrets of the G-Spot Power and his latest which is a Sensual Guide for Goddesses: Sex Woman First: Teach him how You come first. Jean-Claude Carvill conducts a seminar in Los Angeles occasionally. Jean-Claude has also conducted intimate gatherings for women throughout Australia, Bali, France, Beverly Hills, Chicago and Atlanta.

Books coming soon:
The Sacred Yoni of an Escort   **She is a prostitute, bind and frigid**

Available online at Amazon or email jeanclaudecarvillbooks.com

Enquiry: jeanclaudecarvill@yahoo.com

Made in the USA
Middletown, DE
15 July 2018